中医药文化博大精深，
中医典籍卷帙浩繁，
我们从中医药发展的源头开始，
选择极具代表性的节点性事件和重要人物，
结合其在中医历史长河中的贡献与地位
一并介绍，有助于了解中医药发展全貌。

3

Chinese medical culture is extensive and profound with numerous ancient books and records. Starting from the source of TCM development, we select the most representative node events and important figures, introducing them together with their contributions and roles in the long history of TCM, which is conducive to the overall grasp of the development history of TCM.

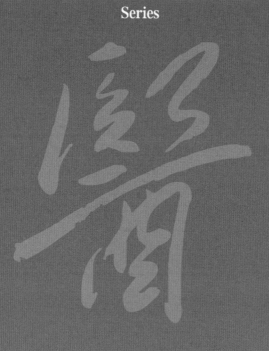

中　医

智 慧 与 健 康 丛书

TCM

Wisdom and Health

Series

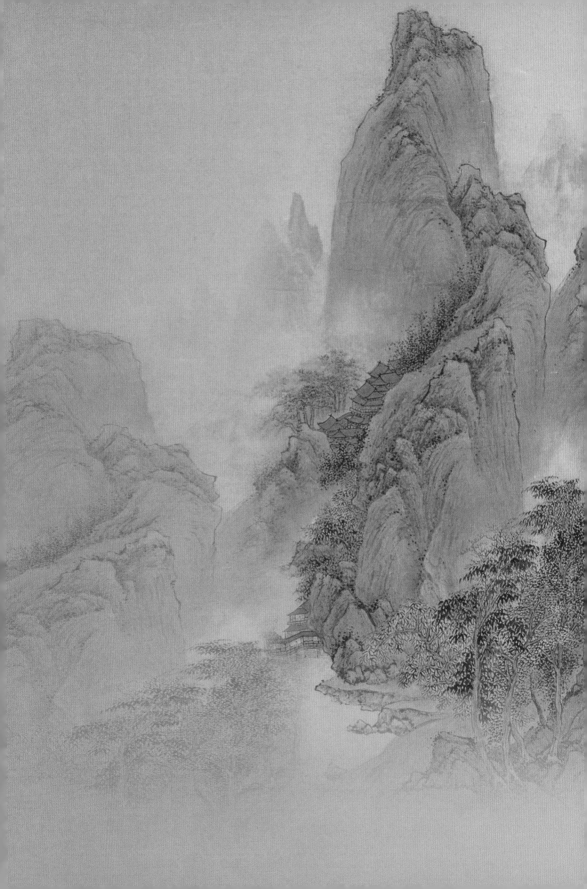

# 中医史话
（汉英对照）

# Historical Narratives of TCM

主　编　王笑频　尹　璐　徐　荣

副主编　黄　达

编　委　（按姓氏笔画排序）

　　　　王桂彬　王笑频　尹　璐　刘　巍　李　奕
　　　　张曦元　恩格尔　徐　荣　高　昂　黄　达

**Chief Editors**
Wang Xiaopin　Yin Lu　Xu Rong

**Associate Editor**
Huang Da

**Editorial Board**
(Listed in order of surname stroke)
Wang Guibin　Wang Xiaopin　Yin Lu　Liu Wei　Li Yi
Zhang Xiyuan　En Geer　Xu Rong　Gao Ang　Huang Da

人民卫生出版社
PMPH　PEOPLE'S MEDICAL PUBLISHING HOUSE

**图书在版编目（CIP）数据**

中医史话：汉英对照 / 王笑频，尹璐，徐荣主编
. —北京：人民卫生出版社，2024.3
（中医智慧与健康丛书）
ISBN 978-7-117-35742-5

Ⅰ.①中⋯　Ⅱ.①王⋯②尹⋯③徐⋯　Ⅲ.①中国医
药学 – 医学史 – 汉、英　Ⅳ.①R–092

中国国家版本馆 CIP 数据核字（2024）第 006823 号

| | | |
|---|---|---|
| 人卫智网 | www.ipmph.com | 医学教育、学术、考试、健康，购书智慧智能综合服务平台 |
| 人卫官网 | www.pmph.com | 人卫官方资讯发布平台 |

---

中医史话（汉英对照）
Zhongyi Shihua（Han–Ying Duizhao）

---

主　　编：王笑频　尹　璐　徐　荣
出版发行：人民卫生出版社（中继线 010-59780011）
地　　址：北京市朝阳区潘家园南里 19 号
邮　　编：100021
E - mail：pmph @ pmph.com
购书热线：010-59787592　010-59787584　010-65264830
印　　刷：北京华联印刷有限公司
经　　销：新华书店
开　　本：710 × 1000　1/16　印张：13.5
字　　数：264 千字
版　　次：2024 年 3 月第 1 版
印　　次：2024 年 4 月第 1 次印刷
标准书号：ISBN 978-7-117-35742-5
定　　价：118.00 元

**打击盗版举报电话：010-59787491　E-mail：WQ @ pmph.com**
**质量问题联系电话：010-59787234　E-mail：zhiliang @ pmph.com**
**数字融合服务电话：4001118166　E-mail：zengzhi @ pmph.com**

# 序

　　中医药蕴含着数千年来中华民族治病疗疾、养生保健的智慧，护佑着中华儿女生生不息，是中华民族的伟大创造与中国古代科学的瑰宝。《中医智慧与健康丛书》正是为了系统总结中医药千年来的实践经验与临床智慧、科学普及中医药知识所编撰。

　　本丛书由中国中医科学院广安门医院牵头撰写，依托国家中医药管理局国际合作司中医药国际合作专项，通过《中医史话》《中华本草》《中医诊疗》《中医养生》四个分册，全方位展示了中医药历史传承、特色优势和优秀成果，旨在向国内外读者普及中医药文化，促进中医药文化的国际传播，做好文明互鉴。丛书精心选取内容，语言通俗易懂，图文并茂，采用中英双语对照的形式，以方便国内外读者阅读。

　　我们真诚地希望通过本丛书，广大读者朋友能够更好地了解中医、用上中医、爱上中医，成为中医的"粉丝"。

《中医智慧与健康丛书》编委会

2023 年 6 月

*TCM Wisdom*

*and*

*Health Series*

# Foreword

Traditional Chinese medicine (TCM) contains the wisdom of the Chinese nation in treating diseases and maintaining health for thousands of years, and protects the endless survival of the Chinese people. It is the great creation of the Chinese nation and the treasure of ancient Chinese science. The *TCM Wisdom and Health Series* is compiled to systematically summarize the practical experience and clinical wisdom of TCM and popularize the knowledge of TCM.

This series is compiled under the leadership of Guang'anmen Hospital of China Academy of Chinese Medical Sciences (CACMS). Relying on the Special International Cooperation Project of TCM of Department of International Cooperation of National Administration of Traditional Chinese Medicine, the series shows the historical inheritance, characteristic advantages and outstanding achievements of TCM in an all-round way ranging from history, materia medica, diagnosis and treatment of TCM to health cultivation, aiming to popularize Chinese medical culture to readers at home and abroad, promote the international communication of Chinese medical culture as well as mutual learning among civilizations. The series carefully selects content, uses language easy to understand, illustrates texts with pictures, and adopts the bilingual form of both Chinese and English to facilitate readers at home and abroad.

We sincerely hope by reading this series readers can better understand TCM, use TCM, fall in love with TCM, and become the "fans" of TCM.

Editorial Board of ***TCM Wisdom and Health Series***

June 2023

# 前 言

中医药学包含着中华民族几千年的健康养生理念及实践经验，是中华民族的伟大创造，对世界文明进步产生了积极影响。随着社会经济的迅速发展，国际交往的广度和深度日益加深，传统中医药学正加快步伐走向世界，被越来越多的国家和地区接受。

为了让更多的人了解中医药、认识中医药，普及中医药健康养生理念，弘扬中医药传统文化，促进中西医交流互鉴，更好地维护人民健康，我们选取了中医药发展史上各时期具有代表性的人物和事件，编成《中医史话》一书。

本书特点如下：

1. **以故事呈现，通俗易懂、有趣有味。**鉴于读者的不同文化背景，以及初学者对专业术语理解上的难度，我们主要以讲故事的方法，图文并茂，对中医人物、中医典籍、中医事件进行解读，可读性强。

2. **以时间为轴，通观古今、采英撷华。**中医药文化博大精深，中医典籍卷帙浩繁，我们从中医药发展的源头开始，选择极具代表性的节点性事件和重要人物，结合其在中医历史长河中的贡献与地位一并介绍，有助于了解中医药发展全貌。

3. **以实用为要，深入浅出、读则获益。**书中选取的案例背后均蕴藏着一定的中医思维和科学方法。如"中医理论基石——《黄帝内经》"中提到的"天人相应"和"治未病"思想，强调人与自然的和谐统一以及早期防治的重要性，时至今日仍然具有很强的现实指导意义。

全民同享健康，世界共享健康。本书旨在普及中医药知识、传播中医药文化，可作为国际友人走近中医、认识中医、了解中医的普及类读物，也可作为初学中医人员整体认知中医、领会中医思维的启发性读物。

本书的编写得到了国家中医药管理局的大力支持，在此深表谢意。我们真心希望通过努力，为各位朋友学中医、用中医、享中医略尽绵薄之力。书中不妥之处，恳请广大读者批评指正。

《中医史话》编写委员会

2023 年 6 月

# Preface

Traditional Chinese medicine (TCM) contains thousands of years' health cultivation philosophy and practical experience of the Chinese nation, which are great creations of the Chinese nation and has had positive effects on the progress of world civilization. With the rapid development of the society and economy, the international exchange is deepening day by day both in breadth and depth. As a result, TCM is going global with an accelerated pace and is being accepted by more and more countries and regions.

In order to make more people learn and understand TCM, popularize the TCM philosophy of health cultivation, carry forward TCM culture, promote the exchange and mutual learning between Chinese and Western medicine, and better safeguard people's health, we select representative figures and events of different periods in the development history of TCM, and compiled the book *Historical Narratives of TCM*.

The features of this book are as follows:

**1. The content is presented in the form of stories, which is easy to understand and interesting to read.** Considering readers' different cultural backgrounds and beginners' difficulty in understanding technical terms, we mainly interpret TCM doctors, classics and events by telling stories with pictures and texts, which is highly readable and memorable.

**2. The timeline is taken as the axis to review throughout the ancient and modern times, and select the fine culture.** Chinese medical culture is extensive and profound with numerous ancient books and records. Starting from the source of TCM development, we select the most representative node events and important figures, introducing them together with their contributions and roles in the long history of TCM, which is conducive to the overall grasp of the development history of TCM.

**3. Practicality is taken as the key, profound theories are explained in simple language and benefits are obtained once reading is started.** There are certain TCM ways of thinking and scientific methods behind the selected cases in the book. For example, the thoughts of "correspondence between man and universe" and "preventive treatment of disease" mentioned in "The Cornerstone of TCM Theory——*Huangdi's Cannon of Inner Classic*" emphasize the harmonious unity between man and nature and the importance of early prevention and treatment, which still have a strong practical guiding significance even today.

Health is shared by all people in the world. This book aims to popularize knowledge and culture of TCM. It can be used as a popular reading material for foreign friends to approach, know and understand TCM, and can also be as an enlightening reading material for beginners to have an overall knowledge of TCM and understand the thinking of TCM.

The compilation of this book has received strong support from the National Administration of Traditional Chinese Medicine, which is highly appreciated here. We sincerely hope that through our efforts, we can help you to learn, use and enjoy TCM. Readers are expected to criticize and correct anything wrong in the book.

Editorial Board of
*Historical Narratives of TCM*
June 2023

目 录

Contents

目 录

Contents

Contents

Contents

# 目　录

Contents

# 中医史话

（汉英对照）

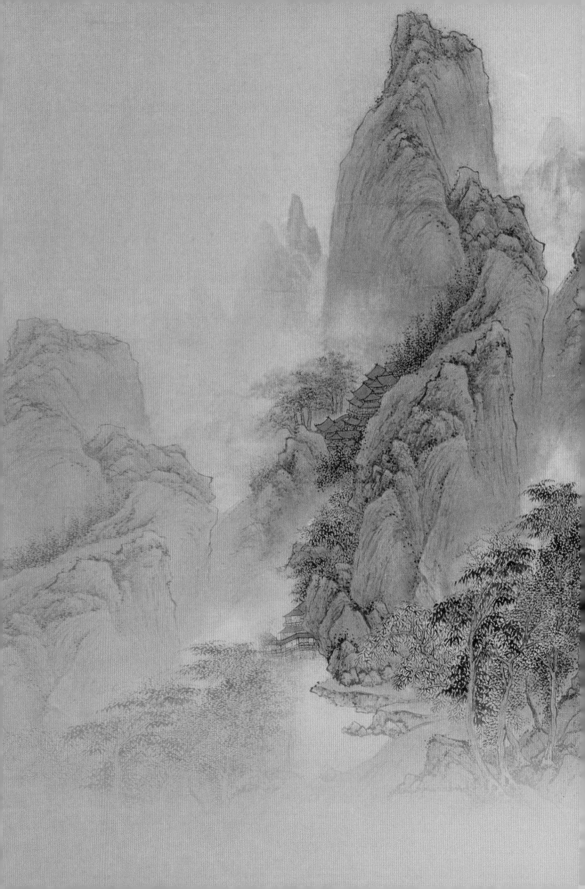

第一章

中医药的起源与理论形成

在中国历史上，关于中医药的起源有很多传说，这些在中国口耳相传数千年的故事，有些带有很浓厚的神话色彩，这些故事和传说反映了中国古代人民在生活生产实践中谋求生存、不断探索和总结与疾病作斗争的经验，以及积累形成的原始医药卫生知识。在这个这漫长的历史过程中，诞生了最早的中医药学理论代表人物及代表著作，这些宝贵的经验为后来中医理论体系的建立奠定了重要基础。

## 一、神农与百草

神农是传说中上古时期姜姓部落的首领，他生活在距今五六千年前的黄河流域，是华夏太古三皇之一的地皇。神农发明了刀耕火种，创造了两种翻土农具，教导部落人民垦荒种植粮食作物并制造出了饮食用的陶器和炊具，因此，被后世认为是农耕文化的创始人，被尊称为"五谷先帝""神农大帝"等。

神农尝百草而创立药物学的传说从上古一直流传至今。《淮南子·修务训》中就有神农"尝百草之滋味，识水泉之甘苦……当此之时，一日而遇七十毒"的记载。《史记》也有"……神农氏。于是作蜡祭，以赭鞭鞭草木，始尝百草，始有医药"之说。上古时期，人类的生存环境非常恶劣，神农对百姓的疾病感同身受，亲自尝遍百草，体察植物寒、温、平、热的药性，并记录下来用来为百姓治病。传说他的身体是透明的，五脏六腑清晰可见，可以看到吃下去的植物在身体里的情况，所以能辨别植物中能够治病救人的品种。神农誓要尝遍百草，解除百姓疾苦。相传他曾在一天之内尝过七十种毒物，曾多次中毒。后来终因尝断肠草中毒而逝世。人们为了纪念神农的恩德和功绩，奉他为"药王神"。客观上说，原始农业兴起后，为寻找更好的农作物种类，人们会更加注意植物的特性，需要了解食物是否有毒、是否可食用，区分植物的不同部位的味道以及植物的功效，在此基础上逐渐形成医药概念，开始医学探索。可以说，医药概念是在人们日常生活过程中形成的，是一种"无心插柳柳成荫"式的发明，这也大致反映了神农尝百草传说的历史原貌。

神农尝百草的传说和故事反映出人们发现和认识药物的实践过程，从中我们也可以推测，来自劳动、生产、生活中的实践经验是中医药发展的源头。古人"医源于圣"的观点反映了上古不同氏族群体在和疾病斗争的实践中对医药经验的积累和贡献，神农、黄帝即是这些氏族群体的代表，这也反映了人们对在医药发展过程中有杰出贡献人物的尊崇。

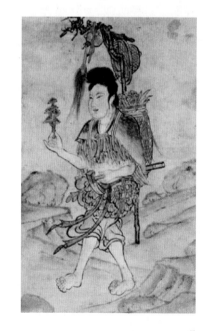

神农像

（1974 年于山西密县佛宫寺木塔内发现，据考证系绘于辽代）

5

## 二、伏羲与八卦

伏羲氏是我国古籍中记载的最早的三皇之一，是中国最早的有文献记载的创世神之一。《三皇本纪》记载伏羲"有圣德，仰则观象于天，俯则观法于地"。关于伏羲这个姓名，历史上并没有准确的记载，有的人认为他姓伏，有的人则认为他姓风，伏羲所处时代约为新石器时代中晚期，是一个蛮荒时代，伏羲发明了钻木取火的方法，给人们带来温暖和光明，极大地改善了百姓的生存条件，百姓非常敬佩和感激他，将他奉为皇帝。

远古时代，人们对自然界的各种现象一无所知，比如刮风下雨、电闪雷鸣，人们不知道原因，既感到困惑，又心生恐惧。为了搞清楚这些自然现象产出的原因，伏羲仰观天，俯观地，废寝忘食地琢磨钻研，连飞禽走兽的脚印和动物身上的纹理都细细研究。《尚书·周书·顾命》伪孔安国传曰："伏羲王天下，龙马出河，遂则其文以画八卦。"这段文字记载的即是伏羲观龙马而画八卦的故事。上古时代，在今洛阳市境内的黄河支流中，出现一头形似骆驼，左右生翼，马身龙鳞，高八尺五寸的海兽。这头海兽在惊涛骇浪中临波行走，人们看其如龙似马，就叫它为"龙马"。龙马的背上背负着河图，上面的斑点规则、美丽，细看是左三八、右四九、中五十、后一六。伏羲听说后特地前来观看，心有所感，于是在甘肃天水的八卦台画出了最初的八卦。八卦是中国最早的文字符号，里面融合了阴阳、五行的原理，是用来推演世界空间和时间的工具。伏羲八卦又称先天八卦，后世周文王在八卦的基础上推演 64 卦，也就是我们今天耳熟能详的《易经》。西晋时期著名的医学家、文学家皇甫谧在《帝王世纪》记载："伏羲画八卦……百病之理，得以有类。"后世据此推断，伏羲在中医的发展过程中发挥了开创性的重要作用。

八卦的发明和传播，使古人在远行时不再因为无法记住来路而迷失。他们凭八卦圭表和几颗较亮的星星就能解决方向难题。为了纪念伏羲发明八卦的伟大功绩，后人将八卦叫作"伏羲八卦"，把龙马出没的河道叫图河。

## 三、《诗经》里的中医药

　　《诗经》是我国最早的诗歌总集，创作于西周初期至春秋中叶，因其优美的韵律、真挚的情感、唯美的意境，在中国传唱千年，是家喻户晓的国学经典。《诗经》反映了从西周到春秋时期农耕、蚕桑、采摘、纺织、染色、建筑、畜牧等人民社会生活的各个方面，同时书中还记录了很多与医药相关的内容，在一定程度上反映了当时的医学发展水平。

　　《诗经》的 305 篇中，有 144 篇涉及植物，记录的植物种类达 50 余种，其中对一些植物的采集季节、产地亦有所记载。虽然书中很少有直接用药物治疗疾病的记述，但从诗篇的字里行间里透露出许多中医药与古人生活相关的记录。如《国风·卫风·伯兮》所写"焉得谖（xuān）草？言树之背"，诗中记载谖草能舒畅情志，令人忘忧，谖草就是我们今天所指的萱草。又如《国风·周南·芣苢》是一首农妇们采集芣苢时唱的山歌，"采采芣苢，薄言采之"中之芣苢即是车前草。其全草和种子均作药用。车前子甘淡而寒，利水通淋。在商周至汉晋时期，医家多认为车前子有强阴益精，令人得子的功效。

　　《诗经》中还蕴含着朴素的中医养生观。在原始的农耕社会，人们的衣食住行在很大程度上都依赖于自然界的赐予，因此古人对自然充满了敬畏之心，在日常生活中也逐渐积累了顺应自然的丰富经验。"天人合一""顺应自然"的养生观点在《诗经》中已有体现。如《豳风·七月》载"七月流火，九月授衣……四月秀葽，五月鸣蜩。八月其获，十月陨萚……"按照一年十二个月的顺序介绍了古人日常生活和劳作时按时节进行的情况，展现了人与自然和谐相处的画面。书中还有古人在饮食中的审美和追求，如《商颂·烈祖》中记载"亦有和羹，既戒既平"。"和羹"是调和羹汤之意，"戒"是指和羹必备的五味，"平"是指羹的味道要平和，体现了古人"以和为美"的饮食养生观，对后世的养生理论有着深远的影响。

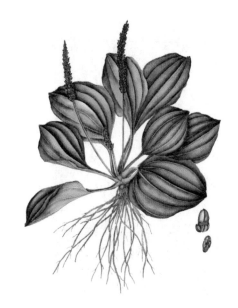

车前草

## 四、中医理论基石——《黄帝内经》

《黄帝内经》是中国现存最早的理论比较完整的医学著作，也是中医传统四大经典著作之一。黄帝，号轩辕氏，为《史记》中的五帝之首，是传说中远古时期的神话人物。他统一了中原，教导百姓播种五谷，兴文字，作干支，制乐器，是中华民族的先祖。《黄帝内经》虽以黄帝冠名，但可能并非为黄帝所撰。因黄帝是华夏始祖，对华夏文明发展产生过重大影响，故后世学者借黄帝之名以提高论著的权威性。现代学者多认为《黄帝内经》并非由一人所撰，而是多个朝代、多名医家的经验和理论总结。

《黄帝内经》最早见载于《汉书·艺文志》，包括《素问》和《灵枢》两部分。原书各 9 卷，每卷 9 篇，各为 81 篇，合计 18 卷 162 篇，内容涉及人体的生理、解剖、病理、诊断、治疗原则、疾病预防等。《素问》内容偏重中医人体生理病理、疾病治疗的基本理论，而《灵枢》则偏重于针灸理论、经络学说、人体解剖等。《黄帝内经》对后世影响极大，时至今日仍是中华文化的象征。其主要成就有 3 个方面：第一，引入了天人相应、阴阳五行学说，从人体本身的整体性和人与自然的统一性两方面，系统而完整地诠释了中医学整体观；第二，论述了解剖与血液循环概念；第三，强调早期治疗的疾病预防思想，中医"治未病"的思想即来源于《黄帝内经》。

《黄帝内经》是对自伏羲、神农、黄帝时代以来至秦汉时期中医药理论的全面总结，是我国现存最早、比较全面系统阐述中医学理论体系的古典医学巨著。它标志着中医学由经验的积累上升到理论总结阶段，完成了中医学理论体系的初步建构。直到今天，仍然有效地指导着中医的理论发展和临床实践。《黄帝内经》作为中国传统文化的经典之作，不仅是医学巨著，更是一部博大精深的文化巨著。它以生命为中心，论述了天、地、人之间的相互联系，讨论和分析了医学最基本的命题——生命规律，并创建了相应的理论体系和防治疾病的原则和技术，包含哲学、政治、天文等多学科的丰富知识，是一部围绕生命问题而展开的百科全书。

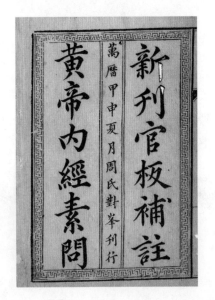

《黄帝内经素问》书影
（现藏于中国中医科学院图书馆）

## 五、第一部药学专著——《神农本草经》

《神农本草经》简称《本经》《本草经》，是我国药物学的第一次系统总结，是中医四大经典著作之一，是已知最早的中药学著作。关于它的成书年代，说法不一。相传起源于神农氏，医史学家多认为该书成书于东汉时期。如同《黄帝内经》冠以黄帝之名一样，书名冠以"神农"，一是因为自古就有"神农尝百草"而发现药物的传说，二是一种尊古风气的反映。

《神农本草经》是对中国中医药的第一次系统总结。全书共分3卷，载药365种，以三品分类法，分上、中、下三品。森立之所辑《神农本草经·序录》说："上药一百二十种为君，主养命以应天，无毒，多服久服不伤人，欲轻身益气不老延年者，本上经；中药一百二十种为臣，主养性以应人，无毒有毒，斟酌其宜，欲遏病补虚羸者，本中经；下药一百二十五种为佐使，主治病以应地，多毒，不可久服，欲除寒热邪气破积聚愈疾者，本下经。"

《神农本草经》中的大部分中药学理论和配伍规则以及提出的"七情和合"原则在几千年的用药实践中发挥了巨大作用，是中医药药物学理论发展的源头。从该书对各种药物的记述内容来分析，主要涉及药物正名、异名、产地、生长环境、采收、贮藏、加工炮制、辨伪、质量鉴别、分类、性味、功效、主治、宜忌、用法，药物的配伍应用规律，方剂的君臣佐使、组方原则等诸多内容，基本上构建起中药学的理论框架。它的问世标志着中药学理论体系初步构建形成。书中记载的药物性味、功效、主治及临床用药理论和原则一直有效地指导着中医临床实践，为后世民众的医疗保健发挥了积极的作用。但限于当时的历史条件，《神农本草经》也存在着某些错误。东汉时期的谶纬神学和道教追求"仙道"的思想就直接或间接地影响到该书，如书中记载"雄黄……炼食之，轻身神仙""水银……久服，神仙不死"之类，曾对后世药物学的发展产生过消极的影响。

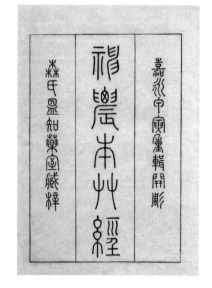

《神农本草经》书影

（现藏于中国中医科学院图书馆）

## 六、中医理论的津梁之作——《难经》

《黄帝八十一难经》简称《难经》或《八十一难》，是继《黄帝内经》之后的又一部中医理论性著作。书名中的"难"字，诠释有二：一为内容深奥难懂，如南宋晁公武《都斋读书后志》说："采《黄帝内经》精要之说，凡八十一章，以其理趣深远，非易了，故名《难经》。"二为问难，即皇甫谧《帝王世纪》说："问难八十一，为《难经》。""经"乃指《黄帝内经》，即问难《黄帝内经》。《难经》与《黄帝内经》虽然没有必然的医学知识传承关系，但它与《黄帝内经》共同构建了中医理论体系的基础，在中医学理论的形成与发展中具有十分重要的作用。

《难经》以阐释和发挥《黄帝内经》要旨为主，其内容和体例以假设问答、解释疑难的方式编纂而成，讨论了 81 个医学理论问题。全书内容简要，辨析精微，内容涉及人体生理、病理和疾病的诊断、治疗等方面，其中尤为突出的是对针灸内容的论述，81 难中有 32 难均有涉及。

《难经》既有对《黄帝内经》精义的剖析疑义，也有对中医理论的开创性发挥，可谓补《黄帝内经》之所未发，扩前圣而启后贤，对后世中医学理论的发展产生了深远的影响。书中记载"独取寸口"的诊脉法、三焦命门理论、针灸补泻方法等，为历代医家所尊崇。魏晋时期的王叔和撰著《脉经》时，就继承了《难经》的诊脉法。此外，《难经》对经络学说、腧穴作用、针刺操作进行了较多的发挥，对中医针灸学的形成和发展也产生了非常重要的影响。因此，历代许多医家重视《难经》，并给予了较高的评价。清代徐灵胎的《〈难经经释〉序》曾评述："惟《难经》则悉本《内经》之语，而敷畅其义，圣学之传，惟此为其宗。"自东汉以后，《难经》一直作为中医经典著作之一流传于世，是中国古代医学家探究医学理论，申明己见，辨证是非的经典著作。

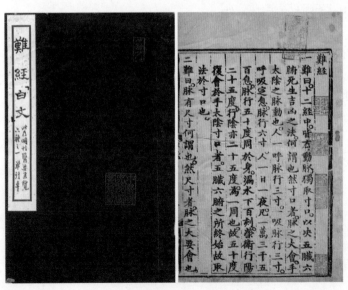

《难经》书影
（现藏于中国中医
科学院图书馆）

# 第二章

# 秦汉、两晋、南北朝时期

——中医药临床实践与学术整理

医学的发展与当时社会政治、经济、文化等诸多因素密切相关。中国历史上的秦汉至两晋南北朝期间，既有皇权高度集中的封建王朝大一统时期，也有战乱频繁、社会动荡的诸侯割据时期。与此相应，中医药的发展既经历了整体提高的时期，也有短暂滞缓的时期。总体来看，历经几百年的发展，中医医疗经验得到不断的积累和丰富，临证领域不断扩大，中医理论得到更多的实践检验，医学体系进一步完善和充实，为隋唐时期中医药学的大发展奠定了坚实的基础。

## 一、神医扁鹊

扁鹊是我国先秦时期影响最大的医学家，也是中国医学史上第一位有正式传记的医学家。关于他的生平事迹，载于司马迁的《史记·扁鹊仓公列传》中。扁鹊姓秦，名越人，战国名医，约生于公元前5世纪。相传远古轩辕时代，人们把一位神医称为扁鹊。因秦越人医术精湛，治病多奇效，人们便把他与远古的神医扁鹊联系在一起，后来干脆叫他"扁鹊"。

扁鹊擅长望、闻、问、切四诊，尤以望诊和切脉著称。据《史记·扁鹊仓公列传》记载，扁鹊仅通过望诊便判断了齐侯的病情和大致的死亡时间，这就是张仲景在《伤寒论》序言中"望齐侯之色"的出处，这反映了扁鹊高超的望诊水平，也说明了他十分重视疾病的预防。他多次劝说齐侯及早治疗，就寓有防病于未然的思想。同时，扁鹊也很精通脉理，尤以诊脉闻名，《史记》中记载，有一次，赵国大夫赵简子骤病，病势凶猛，5天不省人事，赵国群臣非常惊慌。扁鹊为赵简子切脉后认为，病人的血脉正常，并非死症，经过调治，果然痊愈。这个事件充分说明了扁鹊高超的切脉诊断技术。司马迁赞扬说："至今天下言脉者，由扁鹊也。"

扁鹊不仅医术高超，还始终坚持"六不治"的医疗原则，司马迁在《史记·扁鹊仓公列传》中记载他"骄恣不论于理，一不治也；轻身重财，二不治也；衣食不能适，三不治也；阴阳并，脏气不定，四不治也；形羸不能服药，五不治也；信巫不信医，六不治也"。"六不治"的原则反映了扁鹊高尚的医德和反对迷信巫术的唯物主义思想。

关于扁鹊的故事，大多是从民间收集而来，口口相传，难免会有一些误传，但因扁鹊对中医学发展所做出的重要贡献，自秦汉以来，人们十分尊崇扁鹊，各地纷纷为他建庙祠，立陵墓，来纪念这位优秀的民间医生和杰出医学家。

## 二、淳于意与古代医案

淳于意是西汉时期唯一见于正史记载的医学家,淳于意(约公元前215—前150年),临淄人,曾任齐国的"太仓长",所以人们又称他为"太仓公"或"仓公"。据《史记·扁鹊仓公列传》记载,淳于意从小爱好医学,曾拜多位名医为师,司马迁评价他"为人治病,决死生,多验"。

汉文帝四年,淳于意遭人诬告被捕入狱,他最小的女儿缇萦直接向汉文帝上书救父,汉文帝被她的孝诚感动,释放淳于意,这就是历史上"缇萦救父"的故事。后来,汉文帝召见他,详细询问了他学医、诊治疾病、带徒弟等诸多问题,淳于意一一回答。他详尽地介绍了曾经治疗过的25个病人的姓名、性别、里居、职业、疾病、治疗、疗效、预后等情况,在当时被称为"诊籍"。后司马迁将这25例医案录于《史记·扁鹊仓公列传》中,成为我国现存最早见于文献记载的医案。

"诊籍"客观地反映了淳于意的医学思想和诊疗特色。在对病因的认识上,淳于意认为有自然因素,如风、寒、暑、热、水浸等,还有饮食不节、情志过激、劳作过度、起居无常等。如安逸少动可引起肥胖,"得之风,及卧开口,食而不嗽"可导致龋齿等。在所记载的25例医案中,有20例有脉象,其中10例完全是根据脉象来判断死生的。据统计,书中载有浮、沉、弦、紧、数、滑、涩、长、大、代、弱、散等近20种脉象,除了平、鼓、静、躁等几种脉后世未见用外,其他脉象至今还在沿用。在疾病的治疗上,淳于意多采用药物、针刺、灸法等治疗病人,有单用一种的,也有多种方法并用的。这些诊疗方法,对中医理论和临床医学的发展有一定的贡献。

淳于意的"诊籍"既保存了西汉以前医学文献中的有关材料,又反映了西汉初年我国医学所达到的真实水平,并如实记录了他治疗疾病的经验,在我国医学史上具有很高的研究价值,对中医学的发展起到了积极的促进作用。

### 三、外科鼻祖华佗与麻沸散

华佗，字元化，沛国谯县（今安徽亳州）人，是我国东汉末年著名的医学家，与董奉、张仲景并称为"建安三神医"。华佗通晓各种医书，擅长内、外、妇、儿、针灸等科。他的治疗手段多样，处方用药精妙，行医足迹遍及今江苏、山东、河南、安徽部分地区，治愈的病人不计其数，深受广大百姓的热爱和尊崇。

华佗的医术闻名天下，曾给三国时期的许多风云人物治过病，给关羽进行过"刮骨疗伤"，给东吴名将周泰医治过金疮，给广陵太守陈登治疗过内伤。当时的丞相曹操患有头风的毛病，屡治无效，因听闻华佗医术高超，便请华佗为他医治，华佗给予其针灸治疗后，迅速见效。曹操非常高兴，强留华佗做他的侍医，但华佗淡泊名利，不愿自己的医术仅为权贵所用，便托词归家，延期不返。他的行为激怒了曹操，导致他最终被曹操所杀，后世医者无不扼腕叹息。

据史料记载，华佗著有《枕中灸刺经》等多种医书，可惜均失佚。华佗是中国历史上第一位给病人做外科手术的医生。华佗在外科上的杰出成就主要是创用酒服"麻沸散"，在全身麻醉下进行腹腔肿物切除及胃肠切除吻合手术。据《后汉书·华佗传》记载："若疾发结于内，针药所不能及者，乃令先以酒服麻沸散，既醉无所觉，因刳破腹背，抽割积聚。若在肠胃，则断截湔洗，除去积秽；既而缝合，傅以神膏，四五日创愈，一月之间皆平复。"这段文字确切地告诉后人，麻沸散以酒服用，华佗曾熟练运用它做过腹腔肿物切除及胃肠切除吻合手术，大大提高了手术效率，减轻了病人的疼痛。华佗研创的全身麻醉手术，在我国医学史上是空前的，在世界医学史上也是罕见的，其发明和使用完全称得上是世界医学史上的壮举，华佗因此也被后世尊为"外科鼻祖"。我国的历代民众敬仰华佗，纪念华佗的建筑遍及全国各地，如安徽亳州的"华祖庵"，徐州华庄的"华佗庙"，河南许昌的华佗墓地等。

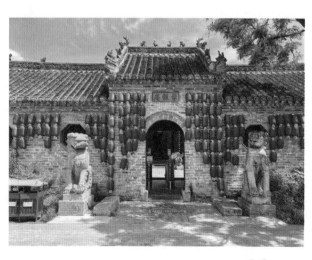

华祖庵

（位于安徽省亳州市）

15

## 四、医圣张仲景与《伤寒杂病论》

张仲景，南阳郡涅阳（今河南邓州）人。他少时资质聪慧，尤好医术，曾拜同郡医生张伯祖为师，经过多年刻苦钻研和临床实践，医术远超其师。后世人因其在中医学上的卓越贡献，尊他为"医圣"。

张仲景生活的年代正值东汉末年，朝廷极端腐败，宦官专权，灾疫连年，百姓流离失所。诸多医者医德沦丧，诊病之时，"按寸不及尺，握手不及足"，"相对斯须，便处汤药"，导致许多患者枉送了性命。面对这样的境况，张仲景"勤求古训，博采众方"，刻苦攻读医学理论文献，参考方药著作，并广泛汲取汉代及以前的临床精华，结合自己长期积累的医疗经验，撰成《伤寒杂病论》。《伤寒杂病论》原书16卷，成书之后，很快因战乱而散失。现今常见的版本是经王叔和整理编撰而成，到了北宋时代又经过医官孙奇、林亿等人的校正，增补成为《伤寒论》和《金匮要略》两本书，前者专论伤寒，对外感热病的辨证和立方用药规律进行了全面概括；后者专论杂病，尤以内科杂病为主。后人将二者称为宋本《伤寒杂病论》。

《伤寒杂病论》是中国医学基本理论和临床实际紧密结合之作，也是我国中医发展史上影响最大的著作之一。它以整体观念为指导思想，以六经辨治伤寒，以脏腑经络辨治杂病，是我国第一部理、法、方、药俱备的医学经典著作。后世的中医名家都非常重视对《伤寒杂病论》的学习和研究，明清之后，对《伤寒论》的研究更成为一个学术流派，影响至今。

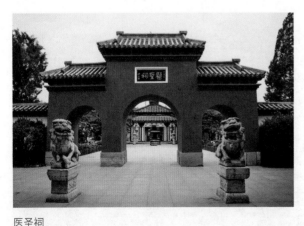

医圣祠
（位于河南省南阳市）

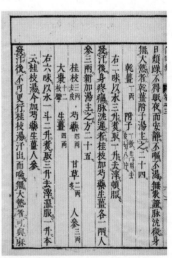

《伤寒论》书影
（现藏于中国中医科学院图书馆）

# 五、道教医学家——葛洪

葛洪（约283—363年），字稚川，自号抱朴子，丹阳郡句容（今江苏句容）人，晋代著名的道教理论家、医药学家和炼丹家。葛洪出身于官宦之家，他一生著述颇丰，但大多散佚。他曾编撰大型医书《金匮药方》100卷，此书已失佚，内容不得详知。葛洪考虑到此书卷帙浩繁，难于携带检索，便将其中有关临床常见病、急症等内容，简编成《肘后救卒方》，后经梁代陶弘景、金代杨用道增补后而成《肘后备急方》，简称《肘后方》，以便临床之需。取名"肘后"即指随身携带以备急用。正由于为救急而作，书中选方务求经典简单，所录药物多为易得、廉价之药，尤适用于平民百姓日常治病急救。《肘后备急方》是两晋南北朝时期重要的医学典籍之一，虽卷帙不多，但内容丰富，也是现存最早的急症诊治专著。

《肘后备急方》是一部以治方急症为主的综合性方书，该书突出了简、便、廉、验的用药特点。书中记载了恙虫病、天花、狂犬病等疾病的治疗方法；此外，葛洪创立的急症治疗技术对临床急症的贡献很大，大大提高了我国古代的急症治疗水平，包括人工呼吸法、洗胃术、救溺倒水法、腹穿放水法、导尿术、灌肠术等。《肘后备急方》中还记载了外伤急救的方法，将开放性创伤伤口称为"疮"，描述了多种伤口止血的方法，并有内病、外发病、各种毒物伤人及虫兽伤等急症的救治法，内容十分丰富。同时，书中还总结了我国晋以来医疗发展的诸多成就，如对疟疾的种类和症状的详细记载，并录有30多首方剂。我国药学家屠呦呦获得2015年诺贝尔生理学或医学奖的青蒿素发明，就受到《肘后备急方》其中所记述"青蒿"治疗疟疾的制备方法"青蒿一握。以水二升渍，绞取汁。尽服之"的启发，可见《肘后备急方》蕴藏着宝贵的治疗经验和医学资料，值得我们进行深入的整理和挖掘。

《肘后备急方》中"青蒿"相关记载
（现藏于中国中医科学院图书馆）

## 六、皇甫谧与世界最早的针灸专著《针灸甲乙经》

皇甫谧（215—282 年），幼名静，字士安，自号玄晏先生。安定郡朝那县（今甘肃灵台）人，后徙居新安（今河南新安）。三国西晋时期学者、医学家、史学家。他出身东汉名门世族，是东汉名将皇甫嵩曾孙。皇甫谧在针灸学史上有非常重要的地位，被后人誉为"针灸鼻祖"。他 42 岁患风痹疾后，开始学医、习针灸，遂臻至妙。皇甫谧参照《灵枢》《素问》《明堂孔穴针灸治要》所叙，"删其浮辞，除其重复，论其精要"，并融合自身实践，无数次以身试针，不断修正完善人体穴位、经脉、针灸医法，撰成《黄帝三部针灸甲乙经》，又称《针灸甲乙经》《甲乙经》《黄帝三部针经》。

《针灸甲乙经》是我国现存最早最全面的针灸学专著。全书共 12 卷、128 篇，前 6 卷论述针灸与穴位基础理论，后 6 卷记录各种疾病的治疗之法，包括病因、病机、症状、诊断、取穴、针灸和预后等。全书采用分部和按经分类法，在总结吸收《灵枢》《素问》《明堂孔穴针灸治要》等古典医学著作精华的基础上，厘定腧穴 349 个，比《黄帝内经》多了 189 个，明确了穴位的归经和部位，统一了穴位名称，区分了正名和别名。同时，采用分部依线法，划分了头、面、颈、胸、腹、四肢等 35 条经络线路，详述了各部穴位的适应证和禁忌、针刺深度与灸的壮数。

《针灸甲乙经》总结了晋以前的针灸学理论和临床治疗经验，为后世针灸学的发展建立了规范，对中华针灸学发展起了承前启后的巨大作用。由晋到宋的针灸著作，如《铜人腧穴针灸图经》，其穴位和适应证基本没有超出该书范围；如《针灸资生经》等专著，无不遵循本书编辑而成；明清两代如《针灸聚英》《针灸大成》等专著，都是在本书基础上发展起来的。该书问世后，一直受到医学界的重视，被作为学医者的必读之书。正如《备急千金要方·大医习业》所说："凡欲为大医，必须谙《素问》《甲乙》《黄帝针经》《明堂流注》……诸部经方。"

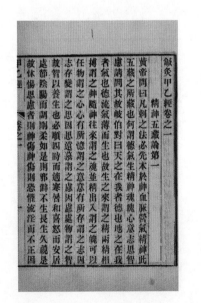

《针灸甲乙经》书影

（现藏于中国中医科学院图书馆）

## 七、王叔和与《脉经》

王叔和，名熙，高平人。生活于3世纪，是魏晋时期著名医学家，曾任太医令。唐代甘伯宗《名医录》言其"性度沉静，通经史，穷研方脉，精意诊切，洞识摄养之道，深晓疗病之说"。王叔和将散在的仲景遗论进行搜集、整理、编次，后经宋代林亿等人校正刊行而流传下来，即今之《伤寒论》。据王叔和自称："今搜采仲景旧论，录其证候、诊脉、声色，对病真方有神验者，拟防世急也。"这说明王叔和对仲景旧论的整理编次是从脉、证、治、方等方面进行的，体现了张仲景的辨证论治精神。

王叔和有着丰富的理论和临床经验，尤精脉学。他在临床实践中深刻体会到脉诊的重要性和复杂性，正如《脉经》序中指出的"脉理精微，其体难辨"。同时又考虑到医者应用脉诊时经常感觉"在心易了，指下难明"，有时甚至将其玄学化，或避而不予考求；已传世的《黄帝内经》《难经》中脉学理论文义深奥难解，脉学专著尚未出现，于是王叔和潜心研究，在总结历代医家经论要旨，载录论脉之说的基础上，结合长期的临床实践经验，终于撰成了《脉经》。

《脉经》全书10卷，97篇，10万余字，是我国现存最早的脉学专著，集魏晋以前脉学之大成。书中将"三部九候诊法"改进为"独取寸口"的诊脉方法，在规范脉名、确定各种脉象特点以及寸关尺分部所属脏腑等方面都进行了系统阐述，使脉法系统化、规范化，极大促进了中医脉学的发展。

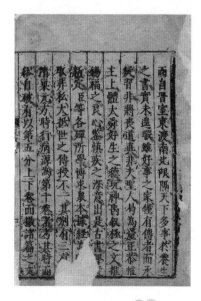

《脉经》书影

（现藏于中国中医科学院图书馆）

19

## 八、山中宰相——名医陶弘景

陶弘景（456—536年），字通明，南朝梁代丹阳秣陵（今江苏南京）人，自号华阳隐居，是我国著名医药家、炼丹家、文学家，人称"山中宰相"。他所著的医学专著有《本草经集注》《集金丹黄白方》《药总诀》等。

梁武帝萧衍未做皇帝前，就和陶弘景是好友。萧衍初夺得大权预备立国，但取什么国号，一时打不定主意。陶弘景根据当时流传的童谣和预卜吉凶的书籍，说其国号应当是"水刃木处"，拼起来是"梁"字，萧衍采纳了他的建议，定国号为梁。事后，萧衍感谢陶弘景，派人进山慰劳，史书上称当时武帝对陶弘景"书问不绝，冠盖相望"。武帝知道陶弘景是个奇才，几次想请他出山做官，但陶坚辞不出。皇帝的诏书催得急了，他就画了两头牛让人带去呈给武帝。画中一牛散放在水草间，一牛则被加上了金笼，有人执着地用鞭子在驱赶它。武帝一看，明白了意思，笑着说道："这人没有什么荣华富贵的欲念，看来是打算仿效在泥淖中拖着尾巴自由爬行的乌龟（语出《庄子》比喻自由自在的隐居生活），哪有招徕的办法？"只是有军国大事，梁武帝仍然派人咨询，"山中宰相"的名声便是这样形成的。

陶弘景对于药物学的贡献很突出，是对本草学进行系统整理并加以创造性发挥的第一人。陶弘景从自己的《名医别录》中挑选了365种新品种附入《神农本草经》，使原书只有365种的药物增加到730种，并予以一一订正、调整、分类注释，编成《本草经集注》一书。他整理时非常认真细心、周密严谨，十分尊重原作，不乱涂乱改，也不信口雌黄，即使有补充也把自己的说法和原书的说法区分开来。他选取的365种药与《神农本草经》合编时，用红、黑二色分别写《神农本草经》与《名医别录》的内容。他开创的这种做法，为后来的注释家争相学习。他首创以玉石、草木、虫、兽、果、菜、米食、有名未用的药物分类方法，沿用至今。经过系统地归纳和总结后，陶弘景第一次提出了"诸病通用药"的概念。这是将药物的功用主治和疾病特点两方面相结合的一种归纳方法，十分切合临床使用。

《本草经集注》的问世，对我国中医药的发展有着很大的影响。我国古代第一部药典——唐代的《新修本草》，就是在此书的基础上进一步修订完成的。

## 九、雷敩与《雷公炮炙论》

中药炮制是随着中药的发现和应用而产生的，其历史可追溯到原始社会。炮制，在历史上又称"炮炙""制造""修治""修事"。《黄帝内经》《伤寒论》《神农本草经》《肘后备急方》里都有关于药材炮制的零散记载。隋唐以前，医生用药多自采自制，后来有了专门的药店，中药炮制也成为专门行业，这就需要制定一套技术标准和操作规范，以保证药效。南北朝刘宋时期，雷敩整理研究前人的各种炮制方法，撰成《雷公炮炙论》。该书是我国第一部较为完整的药物炮制学专著，雷敩因此也被尊称为中药炮制的祖师。

雷敩，生平里居未详，其名最早见于《隋书·经籍志》，又称雷公，于药物炮制颇有研究。《雷公炮炙论》（一作《炮炙方》）共 3 卷，书中载药 300 种，分别介绍药物修事、鉴别、修治和切制、文武火候的掌握、醪醯辅料的取舍和加工炮制方法。此外，还介绍了中药饮片的贮藏、炮制作用及禁忌等基本知识。原书中系统地归纳了"炮炙十七法"，包括炮、炙、煨、炒、煅、炼、曝、飞等常用方法，实用性极强。书中的若干制药方法和选药要求至今仍产生实际影响，被后世奉为中药炮制的经典准则。

《雷公炮炙论》是中国历史上对中药炮制技术的首次总结，也是中药鉴定学的重要文献。原作已经散佚，幸得后世医家著作引用才流传下来。该书对后世药物学发展产生了非常大的影响，明代李中梓《雷公炮炙药性赋》、明代缪希雍《炮炙大法》等著名的中药炮制专著，都是在整理《雷公炮炙论》的基础上，汇集一些民间经验而成。当今中药加工炮制过程仍然参考该书理论，其在提高药效、减缓毒性、调和剂型、方便服用等方面发挥着非常重要的作用。

第三章

隋唐时期

——中医药多元发展

隋唐时期是中国封建社会最强盛的时期，大唐盛世更是中华民族悠久历史中最为辉煌的篇章。这期间，国力强盛、政治开明、经济繁荣、科技发达、文化多元、民族和睦，为中医学的发展和传播提供了良好的基础和条件。中医学在医学理论、药物学、方剂学以及临床各科全面发展的基础上，出现了总结编纂整理的趋势。历史上规模空前的综合性医经方书、集大成的医方著作出现在这一时期，文献整理、药物学著作及临床各科的总结性专著编写水平均有很大进步，对后世医学产生了重要影响。

## 一、最早的国家医学院——太医署

在中国几千年历史发展进程中，隋朝存续时间不到40年，但对中国历史进程和文明发展具有较大影响。隋朝统一了近300年的分裂局面，开创了科举考试，开通了京杭大运河，还开办了世界上最早的"国家医学院"——官办太医署，对后世中医药发展影响很大。

隋炀帝杨广非常重视医学，在他的推动下，隋朝中医学有了新的发展。他在位期间改门下省为殿内省，统尚药局；亲自组织编写了《四海类聚方》（2600卷）、简本《四海类聚单要方》（300卷），对前世医方进行了系统总结。他创立的太医署，既是当时世界上官方最高医学教育机构，又承担了一定的医疗管理职能。《隋书·百官志》载："太常统太医署令二人，丞一人，太医署有主药二人，医师二百人，药园师二人，助教二人，按摩博士二人，祝禁博士二人。"

唐朝沿袭隋制设置了太医署，相比隋朝，唐朝的太医署有了新的发展，一是规模更大，太医署的各类人员近400人；二是分科更细，总分药学、医学、行政3科，每科下根据职能还有细分；三是有明确学制，如内科为7年学制，外科、儿科为5年学制，五官科为4年学制；四是设有专职的管理职位。在太医署的课程中，要求学生对《黄帝明堂灸经》《素问》《黄帝针经》《神农本草经》等中医经典基础课程"皆使精熟"。学生完成基础课程教育后，开始接受专科教育，医学生品学皆优者可提前分配任职，不及格者要降级，且不得超过两年，否则就予以除名。太医署的课程不仅注重经典理论学习，还强调实践操作。课程中还包括中药种植、栽培、采集、存储等内容，要求医学生识百草、懂药性。这种教育模式打破了当时中医教育单一的师带徒模式，培养了很多优秀人才，著名医家巢元方就是太医署的医学博士。

唐朝太医署是世界上最早的医科学校，比欧洲最早的医校——意大利萨勒诺（Salerno）医学校（846年）还早200多年。唐朝政府在中央及各州、府举办医学教育，是我国古代医学教育发展的一大进步，对后世医学教育具有积极的影响。

## 二、第一部病因证候专著——《诸病源候论》

公元 610 年，隋政府组织太医博士巢元方等人编辑《诸病源候论》。该书是中国历史上第一部系统论述病因证候的专著，不仅对秦汉以来临床证候认识进行了全面的整理和总结，而且对各种疾病的病因进行了深入的分析研究，提出许多创见，对后世医学发展产生了很大的影响。

《诸病源候论》全书共 50 卷，分 67 门，载列病源证候 1739 论，它在我国医学上的主要贡献和成就包括以下几个方面：

首先，在病因理论方面突破了前人笼统的"三因"致病理论，丰富了中医学的病因学说。如在书中确认了疥疮等病的病原体，巢元方通过临证观察，指出"疥者，有数种""多生手足，乃至遍体""并皆有虫，人往往以针头挑得，状如水内㿏虫。此悉由皮肤受风邪热气所致也"。由此可见，书中对疥疮病原体及其传染性、发病部位及诊断要点都有比较全面、正确的认识，这比欧洲在公元 1758 年提出的关于疥虫的研究报告早 1000 多年。

其次，巢氏通过长期的实践观察对各类疾病的证候和临床表现均作了详细而准确的描述。如论述胸痹，认为"寒气客于五脏六腑，因虚而发，上冲胸间，则胸痹"，其初期临床表现为"胸中愊愊如满，噎塞不利，习习如痒，喉里涩，唾燥"，甚者表现为"心里强痞急痛，肌肉苦痹，绞急如刺，不得俯卧，胸前皮皆痛，手不能犯，胸满短气，咳唾引痛，烦闷，自汗出，或彻背膂"。书中还对麻风病、中风、黄疸、淋病、糖尿病等疾病的临床表现都进行了详细记载，说明 1300 多年前我国的中医学家对这些疾病就已经有了系统的认识。

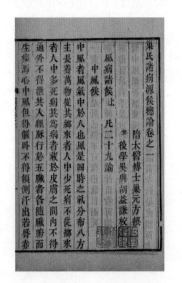

此外，《诸病源候论》中还记载了不少关于治疗创伤的外科手术方法和缝合技术，如在"金疮肠断候"中记述"夫金疮肠断者，视病深浅……肠两头见者，可速续之，先以针缕如法，连续断肠，便取鸡血涂其际，勿令气泄，即推内之"。其中对缝合断肠的理论原则、操作方法及术后的注意事项的论述，至今仍具有参考意义。书中所载的处理腹部外伤、切除大网膜、结扎血管止血、创伤异物清除等技术，反映了公元 7 世纪我国临证医学的重要成就。

《诸病源候论》书影

（现藏于中国中医科学院图书馆）

## 三、药王孙思邈与《千金方》

孙思邈（581—682年），唐代京兆华原（今陕西省铜川市耀州区）人，唐代伟大的医药学家，他天资聪慧，治学严谨，善言老庄，喜好释典，通经史，知百家，是集道、佛、儒三教于一身的饱学之士。孙思邈一生从事临床实践达80年之久，为祖国医药学的发展做出了不可磨灭的贡献，被后人尊称为"药王"。

据《旧唐书》载，西魏大臣独孤信对孙思邈十分器重，称其为"圣童"。孙思邈18岁时立志从医，"颇觉有悟，是以亲邻中外有疾厄者，多所济益"。到了20岁，他开始为乡邻治病，每得良效。从此，他更加勤奋地研读《黄帝内经》《伤寒杂病论》《神农本草经》等古代医药典籍，收集民间流传的药方，寻求民间的治病经验，热心为百姓治病，积累了许多宝贵的临床经验。鉴于古代诸家医方繁杂散乱，检索困难，孙思邈便采集诸家之说，删裁繁复，并结合自己的临床经验，以毕生精力撰成了医学著作《备急千金要方》和《千金翼方》，简称《千金方》。其中《备急千金要方》著成于孙思邈70岁之前，《千金翼方》是他晚年所作，为前者的补充。《千金方》详尽地记载了唐代以前主要医学著作的医论、医方、诊法、治法、养生、导引等多方面的内容，其中汇集的医方计6500余首，载录药物800余种，堪称我国历史上第一部临床医学百科全书。《千金方》的成就，代表了盛唐时期医学发展的最高水平，它不仅在中国影响极大，而且还在亚洲其他国家和地区广为传播，被日本医学界誉为"人类之至宝"。

孙思邈不仅是一位临床大家，而且非常注重医德修养，唐太宗、唐高宗都曾召孙思邈入京都长安并授其爵位，均被他固辞。但当普通百姓求他疗疾时，他却从不拒绝，他强调："凡大医治病，必当安神定志，无欲无求，先发大慈恻隐之心，誓愿普救含灵之苦。若有疾厄来求救者，不得问其贵贱贫富，长幼妍蚩，怨亲善友，华夷愚智，普同一等，皆如至亲之想。"他高尚的医德，一直为后世所称道。他所论述的"大医精诚"观，时至今日，仍是我们进行医德教育时研习的经典。

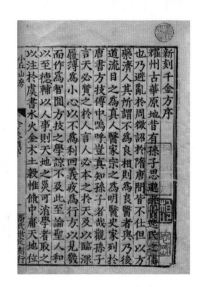

《千金方》书影

（现藏于中国中医科学院图书馆）

## 四、政府颁布的第一部药典——《新修本草》

唐代社会经济迅速发展，交通发达，药物学知识逐渐积累丰富，并出现了许多新药和外来药，本草学知识领域更加扩大。公元 657 年，唐高宗李治采纳苏敬修订本草的建议，征召当时著名的医药学家及行政官员 20 余人共同进行这项工作，并于公元 659 年编纂成《新修本草》。这是我国由政府颁行的第一部药典，也是世界上最早的药典，比欧洲的《纽伦堡药典》（1542 年颁行）早800 多年。

《新修本草》原书共 54 卷，包括药图、图经、本草 3 部分，共收载药品844 种，按自然属性分为玉石、草、木、兽、虫鱼、果、菜、米谷、有名未用 9 类。在此书编写过程中，唐政府广泛地征求各方面的意见，强调"下询众议""定群言得失"。其间，还通令全国各地选送当地所产道地药材，作为实物标本进行描绘。书中的本草部分对古书未载录的药物加以补充，对有误的内容加以修订，并详细介绍了药物的性味、产地、功效、主治及采集时月等。药图部分则是根据广泛征集来自全国各地所产地道药材所绘制的药物形态图。图经部分除了对图谱所绘制的药物形态进行文字说明外，还有药物采集、炮制等方面的内容。

《新修本草》系统总结了唐以前的药物学成就，图文并茂、内容丰富，具有极高的学术水平和科学价值。本书颁行后很快流传全国，当时国家最高的医学府——太医署，立刻将它作为教材。《新修本草》在国外也有较大的影响，该书颁行后不久即传到日本，公元 701 年，日本制定的医药律令《大宝律令·疾医令》就将《新修本草》列为医学生必修书，且学习课时需达到 310 天。《新修本草》原著现已残缺不全，药图、图经部分均已亡佚，仅有本草残卷的影印本和影刻本。因后世本草书和方书对其多有转引，《新修本草》的内容基本上得以保留下来。

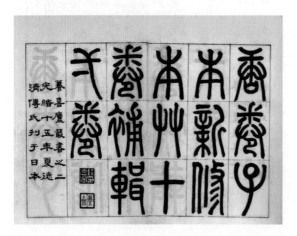

《新修本草》书影
（现藏于中国中医科学院图书馆）

## 五、藏医学集大成之作——《四部医典》

藏医学是中国传统医学的重要组成部分，藏医学的理论体系大约形成于吐蕃王朝时期，即公元7—9世纪。当时的吐蕃王朝与唐朝在政治、经济、文化、医药卫生等领域交往频繁，对藏医学的形成和发展产生了积极的影响和促进作用。《四部医典》（藏名《据悉》）正是在这样的时代背景下由藏族医学家宇妥·元丹贡布（708—833年）所著成。该书是藏医学的奠基之作，为藏医学体系的形成奠定了基础，宇妥·元丹贡布也因对藏医学发展做出的重要贡献，被历代藏医尊为"医圣"。

《四部医典》编写体例与《黄帝内经》相似，以药王答疑形式，采取七言或九言的诗歌体写成，全书约24万字，156章。全书共由4部分组成：第一部分为《扎据》，即《总则本集》，为医学总论；第二部分为《协据》，即《论述本集》，讲述人体解剖、生理、病因、病理，以及药物、器械、治则等；第三部分为《门阿据》，即《秘诀本集》，为临床疾病各论，记载临床各类病症的临床表现、诊断和治疗；第四部分为《亲玛据》，即《后续本集》，补充叙述了脉诊、尿诊，介绍药物的炮制和用法。在《四部医典》成书之后，藏医学家还补充了数以千计的各类小图构成的79幅彩图，对文字内容进行图示，内容包括人体解剖胚胎图、动植物及矿物药物图、各种医疗器械图、尿诊图、脉诊图、饮食卫生防病图等。现存的《四部医典》彩色插图，约绘于明末清初，是我国非常珍贵的医药文物。

《四部医典》对古代藏医理论和实践经验进行了全面系统的总结，反映出许多藏医学的独到之处，是目前保存最为完整且具有很大影响力的传统医学典籍代表之一。它不仅代表了当时西藏最高的医疗水平，也是西藏早期人文、历史、传统、文学、艺术、工艺等的集中体现，并先后被翻译成英文、德文、蒙古文、日文、俄文等多种文字。《四部医典》不仅在当时对世界文化产生了重要的影响，至今仍被认为是极具研究和挖掘价值的重要文献。

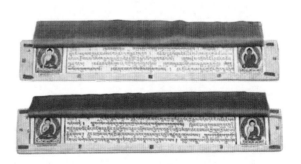

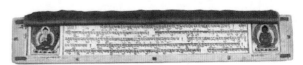

扎塘版《四部医典》内页插图
（刻制于1546年）

## 六、蔺道人与中医骨伤科巨著《仙授理伤续断秘方》

骨伤科在我国源远流长，早在周代就有"疡医"负责处理"金疮""折疡"，汉代军营中已有专门记录官兵折伤的医案"折伤簿"，在各类医籍中也有关于骨伤科医疗技术的论述。唐末由蔺道人所著的《仙授理伤续断秘方》是我国现存的第一部骨伤科专著，在我国骨伤科发展史上具有十分重要的地位。

蔺道人（约790—850年），长安（今陕西西安）人，姓蔺，名失考，唐代医僧。史籍记载唐武宗时曾下诏废佛，下令佛道僧尼26万余人还俗从事农桑生产，收回寺院上田数千万顷，还田于民。蔺道人正是在这种背景下，离开长安，来到江西宜春钟村，并将他的医疗技术和整骨书籍《理伤续断方》毫无保留地传授给一位经常帮他耕耘的彭姓老者。传艺之后，蔺道人另觅地隐居，踪影全无，人们见他忽然消失，便传说他是神仙下凡，将书更名为《仙授理伤续断秘方》。

蔺氏的学术思想源于《黄帝内经》和《难经》的气血学说，继承了《肘后备救方》《备急千金要方》和《外台秘要》中有关骨伤科的经验成就，形成了以整复、固定、活动及内外用药为主的治疗大法，初步奠定了骨伤科辨证、立法、处方与用药的基础，使中医辨证论治原则得以具体运用于骨伤科领域。

《仙授理伤续断秘方》由医治整理补接次第口诀、方论、又治伤损方论三部分构成。书中第一次系统制定了骨折脱臼等损伤的治疗常规，包括局部冲洗、诊断、牵引、复位、敷药、夹板固定等14个步骤，对骨折复位固定，提出了"动静结合"的治则；对复杂骨折的外科手术、手法整复原则和治疗技术进行了详细的论述；在手法整复或手术整复过程中，强调了麻醉药的应用。这些治疗原则和方法至今仍具有较高的理论水平和临床应用价值。

## 七、王焘与《外台秘要》

王焘（约670—755年），唐代郿（今陕西眉县）人，著名医家，是唐朝宰相王珪的曾孙。他自幼多病，常与医药打交道，因此对医学产生了浓厚的兴趣。王焘曾经担任徐州司马和邺郡太守，后至唐朝的皇家图书馆弘文馆任职20余年，因此得以博览方书，采集诸家医方。他所著的《外台秘要》、巢元方所著《诸病源候论》和孙思邈所著《千金方》被后人称为隋唐时期的3部医学代表作。该书博采众家之长，为保存古医籍原貌和总结唐以前的医学成就做出了突出的贡献，在后世广为流传。

《外台秘要》成书于公元752年，全书共40卷，分1104门、载方6000余首，收录内容包括风、外、骨、妇、产、小儿、精神病、皮肤、眼、齿等科，每门记述，先论后方，秩序井然。其中理论部分以巢元方《诸病源候论》为主，医方部分选取《千金方》内容最多。书中整理和保存了大量唐以前的医学文献，所引的资料均注明书名、卷次、便于查核，这种编写体例也为后世医学文献的整理创立了范例。书中收集了大量的民间单、验方，均详述疗效、治疗范围和来源。此外，《外台秘要》对疾病的认识也有新发展，如书中有关糖尿病的记述"消渴者……每发即小便至甜"，比西方威尔斯1670年对糖尿病的认识早了900多年。书中记载的治疗白内障的金针拨障术，是我国历史上最早的记载，至今仍在临床实践中应用。

《外台秘要》成书后很快流传至朝鲜、日本等国，《新唐书》将之称为"世宝"，历代不少医家认为"不观《外台》方，不读《千金》论，则医所见不广，用药不神"，足见该书在医学界地位之高，王焘因此也被誉为文献整理的大师。

# 第四章

## 宋金元时期

——中医药争鸣与成就

宋金元时期是中医学发展迅速、流派纷呈、建树颇多的时期，对后世中医学发展影响很大。尤其在北宋时期，宋太祖、宋太宗、宋仁宗、宋徽宗等多位帝王都非常重视中医，发布了多条旨在发展医药学的诏令。在政府的组织和推动下，各民族之间的医药交流活动频繁，医政设施不断完善，中药学、方剂学、针灸学、临床各科学等发展迅速，官方组织编撰了诸多经典中医药学著作，处方、成药、经络腧穴的规范化研究蔚然成风，在中医药发展的历史长河中留下了浓墨重彩的一笔。

## 一、宋代校正医书局的创办

医政一直被古代帝王作为"仁政"来实施，宋代的统治者非常重视和支持医药学的发展，其中北宋时期发布的医学诏令就有830次之多。如开宝四年（971年），宋太祖赵匡胤发布《访医术优长者诏》，从全国选拔医学人才以充实太医署。太平兴国六年（981年），宋太宗赵炅发布《访求医书诏》，在全国征集医书，按献书多少封以官职或奖赏物资。天圣四年（1026年），宋仁宗赵祯再次征集、校订医书，并令医学家、目录学家予以整理。同时，印刷术和造纸术的进步和发展也为医籍的印刷和传播创造了良好的条件。在这样的时代背景下，宋朝政府于1057年设立"校正医书局"，集中了一批当时著名的学者和医家如掌禹锡、林亿、高保衡、孙兆、秦宗古等，征集、校勘和整理历代医籍。

校正医书局的创立，是我国医学发展史上的一项创举。先后担任校正医书局提举的韩琦、范仲淹等人，都是当时很有影响力的学者。林亿等人在其所校正医书的序文中，多次提当时的皇帝宋仁宗、宋英宗等人对校正医书局的具体要求，如"仁宗念圣祖之遗事，将坠于地，乃诏通知其学人，俾之是正。臣等承乏典校。伏念旬岁，遂乃搜访中外，裒集众本，寝寻其义，正其讹舛""国家诏儒臣校正医书，令取《素问》《九墟》《灵枢》《太素》《千金要方》《千金翼方》《外台秘要》诸家善书校对"。从书中所记述的种种可以看出宋代统治者对医学典籍和古医籍审定工作的重视。

校正医书局设立后，历时10余年，完成了对《素问》《伤寒论》《金匮要略》《金匮玉函经》《针灸甲乙经》《脉经》《诸病源候论》《备急千金要方》《千金翼方》《外台秘要》10部宋代以前最具代表性的医学巨著的校正和印行，为宋代医学的发展和后代医籍的传播做出了非常重要的贡献。

## 二、《太平圣惠方》的成就和价值

《太平圣惠方》是继唐代《千金方》《外台秘要》之后由政府颁行的一部大型方书。书中详尽地记录了北宋之前方书及当时民间的医方，对中医方剂学发展有重大影响，在医学理论方面也有颇多论述和阐发。

《太平圣惠方》由北宋时期的医学家王怀隐奉宋太宗之诏进行编纂。王怀隐，宋州睢阳（今河南商丘）人，初为道士，精通医药，医术高明。宋太宗登基帝位之前，便经常与他探讨医理，宋太宗登基后，令他还俗并任命他为尚药奉御，后升任翰林医官使。978 年，宋太宗诏令翰林医官编纂方书，以官办形式，组织各地名家，从事这项工作。经过全国范围的调研、征集，历时 14 年，992 年终于成书。《太平圣惠方》完成后，宋太宗御赐书名，并亲自制序，足见他对此书的关注与重视。

《太平圣惠方》全书共 100 卷，分为 1670 门，载方 16834 首，包括脉法，处方用药，五脏病证，内、外、骨伤、金创、胎产、妇、儿各科诸病病因证治，以及丹药、食治、补益、针灸等内容。每门之首多载录《诸病源候论》关于病因、病理、证候的论述，并在其后分列对应的方药与疗法。书中强调医者治疗必须辨明阴阳、虚实、寒热、表里，务使方随证设、药随方施；并论述病因、病机、证候与方剂、药物的关系，体现了理法方药较完整的辨证论治体系。所选用的药物品种繁多，而且有些是前人较少使用甚至不用的品种。

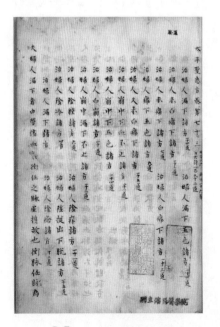

《太平圣惠方》卷帙浩繁，内容丰富，是中国历史上由国家编写的第一部方书。它是一部具有理、法、方、药完整体系的医方大全，对整理和研究中医药学具有非常重要的价值。该书作为宋以前医方集成的巨著，备受历代医家推崇，广为征引，还流传到朝鲜、日本，成书于朝鲜李朝初期的《乡药集成方》，就大量引用该书。

《太平圣惠方》书影
（现藏于中国中医科学院图书馆）

## 三、王惟一与针灸铜人

王惟一（约 987—1067 年），又名惟德，北宋医家，著名针灸学家。曾任医学研究机构翰林医官院医官、殿中省尚药奉御等职，他对古代医籍中有关针灸理论、技术、图经等均有深入的研究。奉皇帝宋仁宗之诏，王惟一整理了前朝书籍中所载有关针灸学的内容，并于 1206 年完成《铜人腧穴针灸图经》。宋仁宗阅后，认为"经书训诂虽精，而学者执之多失"，并指出"传心岂如会目，著辞不若案行"，遂"复令创铸铜人为式，内分脏腑，旁注溪谷，井荥所会，孔穴所安，窍而达中，刻题于侧，使观者烂然而有第，疑者涣然而冰释"。王惟一根据皇帝的要求，于 1027 年铸成针灸铜人两具。这一对针灸铜人当时一是用来作为皇家医院的教学之用，二是用于考核医生针灸技术。

据文献记载，王惟一设计铸造的针灸铜人，一具放置在翰林医官院，另一具放置在大相国寺仁济殿中。铜人身高近于正常成年人，胸背前后两面可以开合，体内雕与真人大小、位置基本相似的五脏六腑。铜人表面镂有穴位，穴旁刻题穴名。空穴由黄蜡封涂，并注水于内（一说注入水银）。若取穴准确，针入而水出；取穴不准，则针刺不入。

相传宋金交战时，金人曾以索取针灸铜人作为一项议和条件，可见其珍贵。元朝定都北京后，将这一对铜人从河南开封移至北京，在 1265 年，由尼泊尔匠人阿尼哥对针灸铜人进行修整。至明朝，明英宗朱祁镇因见王惟一所铸铜人的孔穴经络已昏暗难辨，便组织金工范铜仿制铜人。然而经历代战火之后，宋针灸铜人已经不知所踪。但自宋代针灸铜人问世后，针灸铜人的铸造便由官方向民间发展，明代以后，不断有官方或个人仿制针灸铜人，计百余具。

从古至今，针灸疗法广泛运用于疾病治疗及养生保健中，准确的穴位定位对于针灸的应用及疗效十分重要。针灸铜人作为我国古代针灸教学的模型，对针灸学的发展起到了举足轻重的作用。

## 四、第一部中医儿科专著——《小儿药证直诀》

我国古代对小儿科的研究早已有之，但一直未有全面论述儿科疾病的专著，直至宋代，著名医学家钱乙撰写《小儿药证直诀》，第一次系统地总结了对小儿的辨证施治法，使中医儿科发展达到了新的高度，自此独立为一门专门学科。

钱乙（1032—1113年），字仲阳，祖籍浙江钱塘，后随祖父北迁至东平郓州（今山东东平县）。钱乙自幼丧母，他的父亲钱颢擅长医术，但嗜酒喜游。钱乙3岁时，他的父亲东游海上未返，后来钱乙跟随姑父吕氏学医，精专儿科，勤奋刻苦，博览诸家，闻名于时。宋神宗元丰年间，钱乙去汴梁（今河南开封）行医，誉满京城，因为治好了长公主和皇子仪国公的疑难病症而得到宋神宗的重用，担任太医丞。钱乙在数十年的临床过程中，积累了丰富的经验，他把这些经验和体会结合《黄帝内经》《伤寒杂病论》《神农本草经》等经典医著及诸家学说，写成了儿科专著——《小儿药证直诀》，后经其弟子阎季忠整理总结，核校编辑，于宋宣和元年（1119年）正式刊行问世。该书共3卷，上卷论脉证治法，收列儿科常见病证治80余条；中卷论所治病例23则；下卷为诸方，列载方剂124首。全书论治始终遵循"小儿脏腑柔弱，易虚易实，易寒易热"这一生理、病理特点，遣方用药寒温适度，补泻并用，扶正祛邪兼顾，以柔养脏腑为本。书中详述了钱乙提出的适合小儿用的"五脏辨证"法，记载了钱乙创新的面部望诊和目内望诊方法"面上证""目内证"，即从面部和眼部诊察小儿的五脏疾病的诊断方法。此外，书中记载的许多方剂，如异功散、六味地黄丸、升麻葛根汤、导赤散等，至今仍在儿科临床上广泛应用。

《小儿药证直诀》是中国现存的第一部儿科专著，《四库全书提要》评其曰"小儿经方千古罕见，自乙始别为专门，而其书亦为幼科之鼻祖"。钱乙也因其对中医儿科学发展所做的重要贡献，被尊为"儿科之圣"。

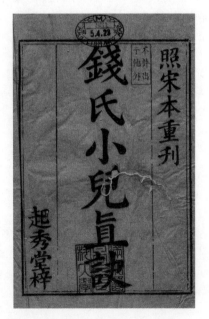

《小儿药证直诀》书影
（现藏于中国中医科学院图书馆）

## 五、解剖新知——《欧希范五脏图》与《存真图》

北宋时期，我国古代解剖学有了重要的发展，此期间前后曾进行过两次人体解剖活动，并由此产生了两部人体解剖学图谱——《欧希范五脏图》和《存真图》。

宋仁宗庆历年间（1041—1048年），广西地方官府处死欧希范等56名反叛者，并解剖死者的胸腹，宜州推官吴简（一作灵简）与医生和画工较仔细地观察了这些尸体的内脏器官，并由画工宋景描绘成图，作成《欧希范五脏图》。《欧希范五脏图》是已知最早的人体解剖学图谱，该图虽早已佚失，难以知其详情，但其绘制过程在许多史志及笔记文集中都有记载，尤其在后来的《存真图》中，对这次解剖活动记载甚详。

《存真图》是宋徽宗崇宁年间（1102—1106年）由医家杨介和画工根据他们所观察到的被宋廷处决剖刳的反叛者的胸腹内脏绘制而成的解剖图谱。《存真图》至清代初期尚存，《文渊阁书目》和《汲古阁毛氏藏书目录·医家类》均有对该图的文字记载。元、明时期的一些医书还转录了其解剖图谱及其说明性文字，《存真图》原稿现在虽已佚失，但其部分内容却由这些医书而得以保存下来。从后世医书的记载中可以看出，《存真图》的绘制十分详细，它不仅有人体胸腹内脏的正面、背面和侧面全图，而且还有分系统、分部位的分图，如：《肺侧图》为胸部内脏的右侧图形；《心气图》为右侧胸腔内的主要血管关系之图；《气海横膜图》为横膈膜正在其上穿过的血管、食管等形态图；《脾目包系图》为消化系统图；《分水阑图》绘出了泌尿系统；《命门、大小肠膀胱之系图》绘出了泌尿生殖系统。所绘诸图及其文字说明与现代解剖学的发现基本一致。

在16世纪以前，人体实际解剖在欧洲极其少见，《欧希范五脏图》和《存真图》的出现及其影响，说明我国人体解剖学的水平，早在11世纪曾处于当时的世界领先地位。尤其是《存真图》，在历史上影响深远，是我国古代医学史上一部最有价值、最有成就的解剖学图著。

## 六、宋慈与法医学大成《洗冤集录》

我国自古重视检验,《礼记·月令》中记载的瞻伤、视折、审断等内容,已可见法医学的萌芽。五代时期和凝父子合著的《疑狱集》(951年)是我国现存最早的法医学专著,此后又有宋代佚名的《内恕录》、郑克的《折狱龟鉴》、桂万荣的《棠阴比事》等相继刊行,不断充实着我国古代法医学的研究。但这类书籍多为案例记载,尚不能认为是法医检验专著,真正堪称我国、也是世界上第一部系统的法医学专著的,当推宋慈所作的《洗冤集录》。

宋慈(1186—1249年),字惠父,汉族,建阳(今福建省南平)人,进士出身,他曾先后四次担任高级刑法官。宋慈一生从事司法刑狱,长期的专业工作,使他积累了丰富的法医检验经验,认为"狱事莫重于大辟,大辟莫重于初情,初情莫重于检验"。他对当时传世的尸伤检验著作加以综合、核定和提炼,并结合自己丰富的实践经验,于1247年著成《洗冤集录》,书中详细记载了人体解剖、尸体检查、现场检查、鉴定死因等内容,并列举了各种毒物的中毒症状,以及急救和解毒的方法。《洗冤集录》与现代法医学相比较,不仅论述的范围和内容基本一致,而且包括了现代法医检验所需要的基础知识,如书中提及用糟(酒糟)、醋等,泼罨尸首及伤痕处,和现代法医学用酸沉淀以保护伤口,防止外界细菌感染,减轻伤口炎症及固定伤口的原理是基本一致的,具有很高的学术价值。

《洗冤集录》涉及生理、解剖、病理、药理、毒理、骨科、外科、检验学等多学科的知识。它不仅是宋代以前法医学成就的总结,而且也从一个侧面反映了我国古代医学发展的水平。该书一经刊行,立即引起全社会的关注,迅速成为当时审案官员的必备书,从13世纪至19世纪,沿用了600多年,后世不少法医书籍也是根据它而作。该书不仅在国内广为流传,在国外也非常有影响力,曾被译成朝鲜文、日文、荷兰文、英文、德文、俄文等多国文字在海外出版,对现代法医学的发展有非常重要的贡献。

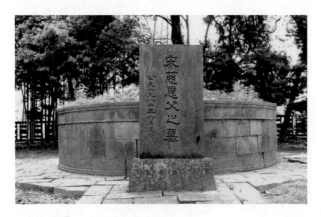

宋慈墓
(位于福建省南平市
建阳区崇雒乡昌茂村)

## 七、金元四大家

唐宋之前，医学领域尚未形成成熟的学术派别，因此医学领域并无学派争鸣的现象。金元时期，由于宋、辽两国以及各民族医药的交流融合，加之战乱频繁，民间疫病流行，给医学研究提出了许多新的问题。在这样的背景下产生了丰富多样的各家学派，形成了百家争鸣的局面，其中最具有代表性的即是被后世称为"金元四大家"的刘完素、张子和、李东垣和朱丹溪。

刘完素（1110—1200年），字守真，自号通玄处士，别号守真子，河间（今河北省河间市）人，故后世又称其为刘河间，其创立的学派为"河间派"。他提出的火热论、运气学说等学术思想对燕赵医学的发展产生了巨大的影响，对后世的补土派、攻邪派、滋阴派、温病派等皆产生了重要的影响。在治法上，刘氏善于应用寒凉药物，故世人又称其学派为"寒凉派"。他首创的"防风通圣散"是治疗表里俱实、清热解毒的良方，至今仍在临床上广泛使用。

张子和（1156—1228年），金时河南人，提出"邪去正安说"。他认为病邪来自外，或从内生，均须以祛邪为主，邪去则正安，不可畏攻而养病。张氏在治疗上对于汗、吐、下三法的运用有独到的见解，尤其注重下法，为"攻邪派"的代表，他的学术思想丰富了中医的病机理论和治疗方法经验，其代表作为《儒门事亲》。

李东垣（1180—1251年），名杲，元时河北定县人，提出"胃气为本说"。主张脾胃健全则不易生病，即使生病也易治愈，在治法上重视调理脾胃和培补元气，扶正以祛邪，于内伤脾胃的理论和治法均有贡献。他的学说对后世医家，尤其是温补学派影响很大，为"补脾派"的代表，其代表作有《脾胃论》《内外伤辨惑论》等。

朱丹溪（1281—1358年），名震亨，字彦修，元时浙江义乌人。他将理学思维应用于医学，将自然界的规律用于人体，提出了著名的"阳有余而阴不足"观点。在治疗上注意滋阴，后人称为"滋阴派"。朱丹溪在金元四大家中生活年代最晚，但他兼收并蓄众家之长，著有《格致余论》《局方发挥》《丹溪心法》等，在中医史上有重要的地位。

这四位中医大家在总结大量临床实践的基础上，对中医理论进行了突破性的创新，以金元四大家为代表的学术争鸣和创新，为中医学发展开拓了新思维、新路径和新方法，极大地丰富了中医理论的宝库，提高了中医药防治疾病的能力，同时对明清时期医学的革新及后来的中医学发展产生了深刻的影响。

## 八、蒙古族营养学家——忽思慧

忽思慧，蒙古族人，生卒年不详，大约生活在13—14世纪。1314—1320年间，他在元朝宫廷任饮膳太医，负责宫廷中的饮膳调配工作，对各种营养性食物和滋补药品以及饮食卫生、食物中毒等均有很深入的研究，是我国古代著名的营养学家。

天历三年（1330年），忽思慧编撰完成《饮膳正要》，该书对元代以前历朝宫廷的食疗经验进行了系统的总结和整理，同时继承了前代著名本草著作与名医的食疗学成就，并汲取当时民间日常生活中的食疗经验。《饮膳正要》以未病先防、重视饮膳、调养脾胃为原则，根据元代宫廷的养生需要、结合当时贵族的饮膳习惯，阐述了饮食养生与保健养生的诸多理论与方法。全书共分3卷。第一卷介绍各种食品，并说明饮食的诸般禁忌；第二卷讲原料、饮食和食疗；第三卷讲米谷、兽、禽、鱼、果、菜、料物等食物的性味、功效、宜忌等，共计230种，其中附图168幅，形象地说明了各种食物的形状。书中还制定了极具营养学价值的食谱，突出强调饮食在日常保健中的作用。此外，忽思慧还特别指明了食疗的应用对象，尤其重视妇幼饮食保健，对妇女妊娠期及哺乳期的饮食禁忌进行了专门的论述，并且增加了不少前代文献中没有记载的药膳方。他对饮食卫生也很重视，对于当时的饮食习惯进行了很多有益的约束，是非常具有现实意义的饮食卫生措施。他列举的许多有效的解救食物中毒的方法至今仍在沿用。

《饮膳正要》是一部融合了蒙汉两族饮食文化的专著。它"将累朝亲侍进用奇珍异馔，汤膏煎造及诸家本草、名医方术、每日所必用的谷肉果菜，取其性味补益者，集成一书"，从营养学角度提出了很多饮食与健康的观点，是我国古代第一部、也是世界上最早的饮食卫生营养专著，具有很高的学术与史料价值，时至今日，依然值得我们进行深入学习和研究。

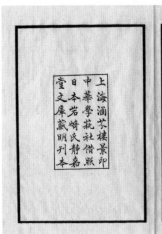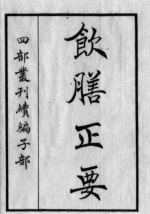

《饮膳正要》书影
（现藏于中国中医科学院图书馆）

# 第五章

## 明清时期

——中医药的鼎盛与革新

明清时期是中医学理论的综合汇通和深化发展阶段，标志性成果是命门理论的发展、温病理论的创新，以及大量的医学全书、丛书及类书的编撰集成，极大地丰富和发展了中医学理论体系，取得了令人瞩目的成就。至民国时期，"改良中医药""中医药科学化""创立新中医"等口号风行一时，这一时期中医药学发展出现了中西汇通的特点。虽然中医药发展并未得到民国政府的支持，但中医药学在民间仍有深厚的群众基础，继续向前发展。

## 一、集大成的医方巨著——《普济方》

方剂是中医学体系的重要组成部分，方书是历代中医文献的大宗。唐宋以来，方书在积累验方的同时，也记录与病证相关的病因、症状和临床各科治疗方法，对方剂的系统理论总结和研究始于宋代，盛于明清。明代集医方之大成者，当以朱橚主编的《普济方》为代表。

《普济方》成书于明洪武二十三年（1390 年）。全书共 426 卷，引历代各家方书，兼采笔记杂说及道藏佛书等，汇辑古今医方。包括方脉、药性、运气、伤寒、杂病、妇科、儿科、针灸及本草等多方面内容。据《四库全书总目》统计，其理论论述共 1960 论，101 门，下共分为 2175 类，计有 778 法，239 图，所收历代医家治疗处方 61739 首，总字数计千万字，在当时的历史条件下，可谓亘古未有之创举。该书采撷繁富，编次详析，是我国现存最大的方书，保存了极为丰富和珍贵的医方资料。

《普济方》所引方书不下 150 余种，其中收录的许多医书现已亡佚。同期编纂的大型类书《永乐大典》素称浩博，此书所引古医籍不见于《永乐大典》者，有 50 余种。《四库全书总目提要》评价此书："是书于一证之下备列诸方，使学者依类推求，于异同出入之间得以窥见古人之用意，因而折衷参伍，不至为成法所拘。"后来学者评价它"古之专门秘术，实借此以有传"，该书的编撰对于辑佚古书，尤其是宋元医籍，具有重要意义。对于今天中医药领域的研究者来说，也可依据此书考证方剂的源流正变，参考异同，具有很大的参考价值。

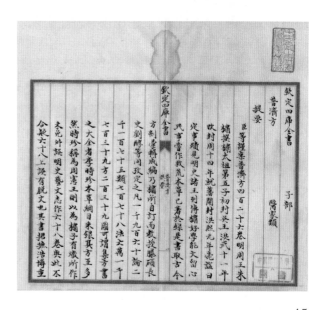

《普济方》书影
（清代《四库全书》抄本，
现藏于中国中医科学院图书馆）

## 二、人痘接种预防天花

我国人痘接种预防天花的文献记载首见朱纯嘏所著《痘疹定论》一书。书中记载：宋真宗时期，宰相王旦的几个子女均不幸死于天花，后老来得子，取名王素。为了避免王素重蹈覆辙，王旦便召集众多名医商议防治痘疮的方法。听闻四川峨眉山有"神医"能接种人痘预防天花，遂请其为王素种痘。王素种痘后第 7 天，全身发热，至 12 天后痘已结痂。其后，人痘接种预防天花的技术历经各代医家的不断实践和完善，逐渐成为中国古代预防天花的主要方法，但这项技术能在后来得到广泛推广和传播，与清朝康熙皇帝的重视密不可分。

明清时期，天花肆虐，据文献记载满族皇室许多成员皆死于天花，当时民众畏痘如虎，遇天花暴发流行期，只能消极躲避。面对这种情况，康熙开始积极寻求天花的预防措施。康熙二十年（1681 年），康熙命内务府馆员徐定弼至江西寻访种痘医师，地方官员李月桂推荐朱纯嘏应诏，经验证方法有效后，朱纯嘏便为皇室和宫廷官员子孙种痘。随后，朱纯嘏任职太医院，太医院由此也设立了痘疹科，专门负责种痘和治痘工作。此后他还被派遣到边外 49 旗及喀尔喀，为满蒙官员的子孙种痘。康熙皇帝在《庭训格言》中曾说："国初人多畏出痘，至朕得种痘方，诸子女尔等子女，皆以种痘得无恙，今边外四十九旗，及喀尔喀诸藩，俱命种痘，凡所种皆得善愈。"由于皇帝下令推广预防天花的人痘接种技术，"经余种者不下八九千人，屈指计之，所莫救者，不过二三十耳。"可见这项技术在 18 世纪中叶已经比较成熟。

人痘接种技术被誉为人类免疫学的先驱，这项技术不仅在当时的中国得到了广泛的应用，而且在世界范围内得到了普及，先传至俄国、日本和朝鲜，后再传至北欧和英国各地，直到 1796 年，英国人琴纳试种牛痘成功，才逐渐被牛痘法所取代。法国启蒙思想家伏尔泰曾在《哲学通信》中写道："我听说一百年来中国人一直有此习惯（指种痘），这是被认为全世界最聪明，最讲礼貌的一个民族作出的伟大先例和榜样。"可以说，人痘接种技术为人类的传染病防治做出了巨大的贡献。

### 三、李时珍与《本草纲目》

李时珍（1518—1593 年），字东璧，晚年自号濒湖山人，湖北蕲州（今湖北省蕲春县蕲州镇）人。他出生于医生世家，自幼习儒，23 岁开始随其父学医，医名日盛。李时珍 33 岁时，因治好了富顺王朱厚焜儿子的病而医名大显，被推荐至太医院工作。这期间，他饱览群书，积极地从事药物研究工作，经常出入于太医院的药房及御药库，认真仔细地比较、鉴别各地的药材，搜集了大量的资料。李时珍结合自己数十年的行医经验，发现古代本草书中存在着不少错误，于是决心重新编纂一部本草书籍。为了完成这个宏伟的心愿，李时珍自 1565 年起，先后到武当山、庐山、茅山、牛首山及湖广、安徽、河南、河北等地收集药物标本和处方，并拜渔人、樵夫、农民、车夫、药工、捕蛇者为师，参考历代医药等方面书籍 925 种，考古证今、穷究物理，记录了上千万字札记，历经 27 个寒暑，三易其稿，于明万历十八年（1590年）完成了 192 万字的巨著《本草纲目》。

《本草纲目》是我国古代最伟大的药学著作。该书集明以前本草学之大成，分类科学、内容丰富，在世界医学史占有很重要的地位。《本草纲目》全书共收录药物 1892 种，其中有 374 种药物为李时珍通过亲自采访和考察后新增的。该书按照"物以类聚，目随纲举"的原则将药物按照自然属性归纳，共设 16 部，在各部之

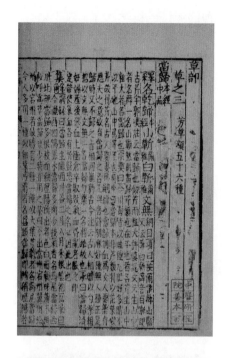

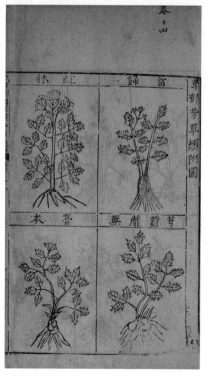

《本草纲目》书影

（现藏于中国中医科学院图书馆）

下又再分为若干类，建立了先进的药物分类体系。书中对药物的记述，涵盖了药物的名称、产地、品种、形态、炮制方法、性味、功效、主治等，对药物品种的考证，科学严谨，议论精详。此外《本草纲目》中还记载了与药物的形态、生态环境相关的自然科学知识。

《本草纲目》的问世，将本草学的发展推至了前所未有的高度。明末以后，该书多次刊行，影响深远。李时珍为修撰本草穷尽了毕生精力。这种锲而不舍、至臻至善的责任心和使命感也是千年来中医文化精神传承的最好诠释。时至今日，李时珍的中华传统医学思想和《本草纲目》丰富的内容对中华传统医学的研究发展及临床实践仍具有重要的指导价值，也越来越受到中外学术界的重视。

## 四、吴又可《温疫论》与传染病理论革新

《黄帝内经》中论述"五疫之至，皆相染易，无问大小，病状相似"，这是我国关于传染病学说最早的文献记载。巢元方在《诸病源候论》中记载了温病34候，更以时行、戾气、伤寒论述了3种不同类型的传染病。明代医家王履在《医经溯洄集》中指出："温病、热病，此以天时与病形而为病名者也。"同时指出温热病是"怫热自内而达于外"。至明末，温病学说逐渐兴起并有了新的发展，其中最具代表的人物是吴又可。

吴又可（1582—1652年），字有性，江苏吴县（今江苏省苏州市）人，明末清初传染病学家，是我国古代温病学说的主要奠基人之一。据文献记载，明代共暴发大瘟疫64次，吴又可亲历了崇祯十四年（1641年）流行于河北、山东、江苏、浙江等省的瘟疫，面对大疫，他愤而发声：大批因疫而死者，并非死于病，而是死于医。他通过亲身观察和诊病施药的临床实践，在继承前人有关温病论述的基础上，创造性地提出了温病不同于伤寒的系统见解，于1642年编著完成《温疫论》，在传统理论的基础上革新发展了传染病学说，开创了传染病研究的先河。

吴又可创造性地提出"戾气学说"，他认为传染病的病因"非风、非寒、非暑、非湿，乃天地之间别有一种异气所感"，即戾气。他还指出了"戾气"的传播途径，认为"戾气"通过口鼻侵犯人体，"自口鼻而入"，而是否致病，既与戾气的量、毒力大小有关，也与人体抵抗力强弱有关，这一论述，科学地预见了传染病的传播途径。同时，吴又可在大量实践鉴别经验的基础上，提出人和牲畜都会因为戾气致病，但是戾气的种类不同，所引起的疾病也不同，"万物各有宜忌，宜者益而忌者损，损者制也，故万物各有所制"。可见，他对传染病病原致病的特异性的问题已经有了比较科学的认识。

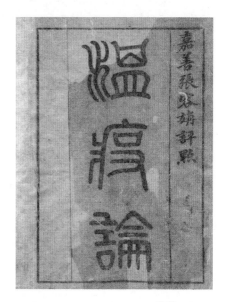

《温疫论》成书后流传甚广，影响深远。在当时没有显微镜观察细菌、病毒等致病微生物的情况下，吴又可就已经科学地预见其存在，并对温病的病因、传染途径等进行了深入系统的论述，为温病学说的系统化做出了巨大的贡献。

《温疫论》书影

（现藏于中国中医科学院图书馆）

## 五、陈实功与《外科正宗》

陈实功（1555—1636 年），字毓仁，号若虚，江苏南通人，明代著名外科学家。自幼精研外科医术，他少年时期师从著名文学家、医学家李沦溟，并深受老师影响。李沦溟认为："内之症或不及外，外之症则必根于其内也。"这也成为陈实功数十年外科医疗生涯的座右铭。他继承和发展了李沦溟的观点，主张外科疾病应采取内治或内治与外治相结合的方法，强调外部手术与内服药物配合使用。

陈实功于 1617 年编著完成《外科正宗》一书，全书共 12 卷 157 篇，对痈疽、疗疮、流注、瘰疬、瘿瘤、肠痈、痔、白癜风、烫伤、疥疮等外、伤、皮肤、五官科疾病，"分门逐类，统以论，系以歌，淆以法，则微至疥癣，亦所不遗"。书中对 100 余种外科常见病症，大多都做了系统的论述，对每类病症多论述其病因病理、症状证候、诊断及治疗方法。在治法上，陈实功主张内外并重，"消""托""补"三法结合，内服药与外治法兼施。在外科手术治疗上，他继承和发扬了截趾术、咽部异物剔除术、下颌骨脱臼复位术、气管缝合术等。同时，他还设计制造了许多简便有效的外科手术器械，如创造乌龙针用于咽部异物取出，用细铜箸进行鼻息肉摘除，对当时外科手术水平的提高具有重要的意义。《外科正宗》对皮肤病、肿瘤也多有论述，对于肿瘤，陈实功认为肿瘤只有及早发现，摸清病源，才能及早治疗，有希望治愈。

《外科正宗》以"列症最详，论治最精"著称，分析详尽，论治精辟，治法得当，反映了明朝以前我国外科学的重要成就。《外科正宗》是中医外科的经典著作。其刊行后，广为传播，并流传到日本等国，具有较高的学术价值，是中医外科的经典著作。

## 六、眼科专著《银海精微》的出色成就

《银海精微》是驰名中外的眼科著作，现在刊印的通行本题为唐代孙思邈辑，今之学者多认为是托名所作，国内学者多认为该书成于明朝。中国的道家以目为银海，故《银海精微》即寓意本书富含眼科理法方药微妙精华之意。该书在汲取前朝眼科成就基础上，补充了多种眼病的诊治方法，将眼科理论和药物、手术治疗紧密结合起来，具有极高的学术价值。

《银海精微》全书共2卷，列有82种病症，主要包括睑生风粟（砂眼）、远视、近视等，其中有80症配有附图，以标示病变部位或病态。书中对眼科手术方法的记述颇为翔实，对劀洗、钩、割、针、烙等手术方法，手术步骤，适应证及禁忌证均有明确记载，对不同原因造成的眼科疾病的治疗难易程度和不同的治疗效果也有涉及，如因肝肾二经病症所引起的血灌瞳仁，强调"此血难退"，对因外伤所造成的血灌瞳仁，则指出"灌虽甚，退之速，手术误伤亦然"。书中记载的这些手术疗法和外治法，有些也是现代西医所常用的治疗方法。此外，《银海精微》在眼科疾病诊断上也有重要贡献，指出在望诊时"凡看眼法，先审瞳仁神光，次看风轮，再察白仁，四辨胞睑，此四者，眼科之大要"。

《银海精微》辨证细致入微，图文并茂，立法平正不偏，选方实用有效，对明代及以后眼科学的发展有着非常广泛的影响，清代《四库全书总目提要》评价它："其辨析诸证，颇为明晰。其法补泻兼施，寒温互用，亦无偏主一格之弊。"书中对眼科诸病治疗方剂、金针拨翳障法、药方歌诀以及眼科常用药的药性的论述，至今仍在中医眼科临床发挥着重要的作用。该书还被西方学者译成英文，在世界范围广为传播。

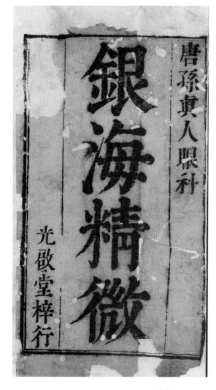

《银海精微》书影

（现藏于中国中医科学院图书馆）

## 七、承前启后的《针灸大成》

《针灸大成》是针灸学著作，由明代杨继洲撰写，靳贤补辑重编，首刊于明万历二十九年（1601年），共10卷。

杨继洲，名济时，明代三衢（今浙江省衢州市六都杨村）人。杨家世代业医，其祖父曾任太医院太医，颇有声望，家藏秘方、验方与医学典籍极为丰富，编纂成家传著作《卫生针灸玄机秘要》，然而此书一直未能刊刻问世。杨继洲幼时博极群书，后弃儒从医，寒暑不辍，因感"诸家书弗会于一"，将家传与诸家医籍之针灸论述，参合指归，汇同考异。恰逢山西监察御史赵文炳患痿痹之疾，多方诊治，屡治不愈，邀杨继洲去山西诊治，先生仅仅针刺了三针，痿痹竟当场痊愈。赵文炳为答谢杨继洲，决定帮助他刊印《卫生针灸玄机秘要》一书，并委托晋阳人靳贤进行选集校正。但杨继洲认为书稿内容仍有欠缺，遂在《卫生针灸玄机秘要》的基础上，结合40余年临床经验，辑录了《医经小学》《针灸聚英》《标幽赋》《医学入门》《古今医统》等20余本明代以前的重要针灸论著，博采众长编写了《针灸大成》这部完备而实用的针灸专著。

《针灸大成》内容丰富，广泛辑录了《黄帝内经》《难经》等古医籍中有关针灸的论述，收录了历代名家各据心得编成的针灸歌赋，重新考证了穴位、经络、历代针灸的操作手法，记载了各种病证的配穴处方和治疗验案。该书有系

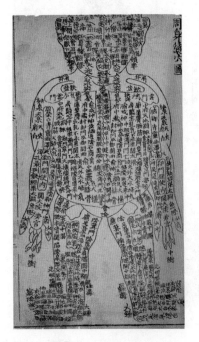

统完整的针灸学理论，融合了众多针灸大家的临床经验，全面呈现了明代以前针灸学发展的脉络，被认为是继《黄帝内经》《针灸甲乙经》后针灸学历史上第三次大总结。此书自明万历年间刊行以来，已被译成英文、日文、德文、法文、拉丁文等多种文字，至今仍存47种版本，平均每6.8年就有新版本问世。其版刻次数之多、流传之广、影响之大、声誉之隆，都是历来罕见的。《针灸大成》的问世，标志着中国古代针灸学已经发展到了相当成熟的地步，后人在论述针灸学时，大多将《针灸大成》作为最重要的参考书之一，在针灸学发展历史上起到了承前启后的重要作用。

《针灸大成》所载人体周身总穴图
（现藏于中国中医科学院图书馆）

## 八、温病学说大家——叶天士

叶天士（1667—1746 年），名桂，字天士，号香岩，江苏吴县（今江苏省苏州）人。清代著名医学家，擅长治疗时疫和痧痘等症，是中国最早发现猩红热的医家。其在温病学上的成就尤其突出，首创温病"卫、气、营、血"的辨证大纲，为温病辨证论治开辟了新途径，是温病学的奠基人之一。

叶天士出生于医学世家，祖、父两代俱业医，少时即受家学，14 岁时父亲逝世，师从父亲门人朱某，此后 10 年间，先后从师 17 人，"闻某人善治某证，即往，执弟子礼甚恭"，吸取各家所长，刻苦钻研，融会贯通，诊治疗效显著，在百姓中有很高的声望。他一生忙于诊治疾病，而无暇著书，现传的《温热论》《临证指南医案》《叶氏存真》《未刻叶氏医案》等，都是其门人根据他的口授或临床实践中的笔记整理编辑而成。

叶天士首先从病因、感受途径和传变规律上对伤寒与温病作出了区分，明确提出"温邪"是导致温病的主因。其次提出"温邪上受，首先犯肺，逆传心包"的论点，概括了温病的发展和传变的途径，成为认识外感温病的总纲；还根据温病病变的发展，创立了卫气营血的辨证方法，指出温病传变的规律，即"大凡看法，卫之后方言气，营之后方言血"。将其概括为卫、气、营、血四个阶段，总结出"在卫汗之可也""到气才可清气""入营犹可透热转气""入血直须凉血散血"的治疗原则。叶天士还详述查舌、验齿、辨斑疹白㾦等在温病诊断上的意义，为温病临床诊断做出了贡献。

叶氏一生中培养了很多济世救人的名医，更留下大量医案，为后世者所传诵。《清史稿》称"大江南北，言医者辙以桂为宗，百余年来，私淑者众"。叶桂在世 80 年，始终保持对医学的敬畏之心，临终前警诫他的后人们说："医可为而不可为，必天资敏悟，又读万卷书，而后可借术济世。不然，鲜有不杀人者，是以药饵为刀刃也。吾死，子孙慎勿轻言医。"

## 九、吴鞠通与《温病条辨》

吴鞠通（1758—1836 年），名瑭，字配珩，号鞠通，清代淮安府山阳县（今江苏省淮安市淮安区）人，代表作《温病条辨》，是继叶天士、薛雪之后的温病学派重要代表人物。

吴鞠通出生于书香家庭，受其父影响，吴氏自幼攻读儒书，希图科名。然在其 19 岁时，父亲久病不愈逝世。在读到张仲景《伤寒论》的序言中"外逐荣势，内忘身命"之后，吴氏放弃了考取功名的念头，转而致力于救人济世。他一生中经历多次瘟疫流行，亲人亦有死于温病者，因而致力于温病学的研究。他认为虽然吴又可的《温疫论》议论宏阔，发前人所未发，但细查其发，未免支离驳杂。而叶天士持论平和，立法精细，但有医案散见于杂症之中，人多忽之而不深究。因此，他潜心研究，结合自己的临床经验，考证《黄帝内经》《伤寒论》等书，结合历代医家对温病的认识，撰写了《温病条辨》一书。此书标志着中医温病学完整的理论体系的形成，是中医学发展史上的重要里程碑。直到今天，在防治温热病方面，仍有重要的参考价值。

吴鞠通首先从根本性质上将伤寒与温病区分开来，伤寒之原，原于水；温病之原，原于火，认为伤寒与温病两病有水火的区别。其次将温病分为九种：风温、温热、温疫、温毒、暑温、湿温、秋燥、冬温、温疟。温疫只是 9 种温病之一，具有强烈的传染性，而其他 8 种，可从季节及疾病表现上加以区分，由此确定了温病学说的研究范围。在温病的病机方面，吴鞠通认为是从三焦而变化的。将温病传变与脏腑病机联系起来，"温病自口鼻而入，鼻气通于肺，口气通于胃，肺病逆传，则为心包。上焦病不治，则传中焦胃与脾也。中焦病不治，则传下焦肝与肾也。始上焦，终下焦"，补充和完善了叶天士的卫气营血辨证。吴鞠通在书中还确立了清热养阴这一温病治疗的基本大法，提出温病不同阶段的治疗方剂：在卫用银翘散、桑菊饮；入气服白虎汤、承气汤；在营施以清营汤、清宫汤；入血则饮犀角地黄汤等。吴鞠通为温病学说理、法、方、药系统的完善做出了重大贡献。

## 十、最权威的中医学教科书——《医宗金鉴》

清朝前期社会经济发展迅速，国力昌盛，宫廷医学也登峰造极。1739 年，乾隆皇帝诏令太医院右院判名医吴谦主持编纂一套大型的医学丛书，以标榜文治从而"以正医学"，"使为师者，必由是而教；为弟子者，必由是而学"。

吴谦，字六吉，安徽歙县人。后人称其与喻昌、张璐为清初三大家。吴谦奉旨后，为了修正医经典籍以及各家医书存在的"词奥难明、传写错误、或博而不精、或杂而不一"等问题，他不仅参考朝廷的内库藏书，还下令征集全国各种新旧医书与经验良方，并且挑选了精通医学、兼通文理的 70 多位官员共同编修，分门别类以去芜取精，博采众长，历时 3 年编辑完成，乾隆皇帝赐名为《医宗金鉴》。1749 年，清太医院将《医宗金鉴》定为医学生教科书，逐步成为全国医学教学标准，在全国推行，影响极为深远。

《医宗金鉴》是一本兼具教学与临床诊治性质的医学丛书，注重实用性，内容深入浅出，全书共 90 卷，15 个分册，内容极为丰富，采集了上自春秋战国，下至明清的历代名著之精义，包括伤寒 17 卷，金匮 8 卷，名医方论 8 卷，四诊 1 卷，运气 1 卷，伤寒心法 3 卷，杂病心法 5 卷，妇科心法 6 卷，幼科心法 6 卷，痘疹心法 4 卷，种痘心法 1 卷，外科心法 16 卷，眼科心法 2 卷，针灸心法 8 卷，正骨心法 4 卷，全书约 160 万字。该书不仅搜集了许多古传药方，而且对名医张仲景的著作《伤寒论》和《金匮要略》作了订正，其目的是"俾二书并行于世，庶后之业医者，不为俗说所误，知仲景能治伤寒，未尝不能治杂证也"。该书是我国综合性中医医书中最完善简要的一种，图、文、方、论兼备，歌诀助诵，适合初学者，同时，讲解详细处可作为医生临床诊治疾病时参考使用，是我国第一部带有教材性质的普及性医学丛书。

《医宗金鉴》有十分明显的时代性，适应18 世纪中国疾病谱，尤其切合临床实用，切实改善了当时天花流行的危害，设立了专门的痘疹科，使理论与技术融合升级，应用极为广泛。此书后被《四库全书》收入，《四库全书总目提要》对《医宗金鉴》有很高的评价。

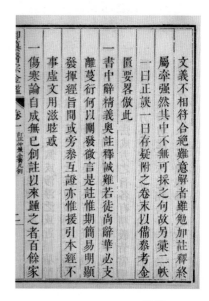

《医宗金鉴》书影

（现藏于中国中医科学院图书馆）

## 十一、外治宗师——吴尚先

吴尚先（1806—1886年），名樽，原名安业，字尚先，又字师机、权仙，别号潜玉居士、潜玉老人，清钱塘（今浙江省杭州市）人，清代著名医学家。吴尚先出生在文学世家，自幼习儒。他从小就受到家学的熏陶，经史子集无所不读，道光十四年（1834年）考中举人，成为候补知县，官至内阁中书。后来因病没有参加京试，渐渐无心于仕途功名，跟随父亲"寓居于扬（州），诗文之外，兼学为医"。从此踏上了"不为良相，便为良医"的道路，精心攻读医学，上至《灵枢》《素问》，下至《伤寒论》《金匮要略》，历代名家医典，无所不读。

1851年，太平天国运动爆发，很快就波及整个江南地区，为躲避战乱，吴尚先和家人避居泰州，并在那里以外治法行医救人。由于当时处于战乱，当地又气候潮湿，农民涉水耕作，痹证的发病率很高，而且血吸虫病等疾疫也很流行，民众因经济和医疗条件的限制得不到及时有效的医治，以致死者颇多。由于药物比较匮乏，吴尚先为了能救治病患，广泛汲取前人经验，创用内病外治法，以疗治薄贴（即膏药）、熏洗等法治疗内、外、妇、儿等科各种疾病，治法简便，疗效显著，应用广泛，所以很受广大民众的欢迎。同治三年（1864年），经过十多次改稿，他吸取前人和古籍中有关外治论述，汇集民间外治疗法，著成我国历史上第一部外治法专书《理瀹骈文》（又名《外治医说》），对中医外治法进行了全面系统的整理与总结，详细论述了膏药的治病机理，指出膏药的配制方法和应用方法。吴尚先生活的时代是"西学东渐"的大时代，西方医学逐步传播到中国，但吴尚先并没有盲目排外，而是在坚持中医为主的基础上吸取西方外治之所长。书中也介绍了西方医学外治的方法，如治吐血、衄血等症，还提到了西方传入的输血法等。此外，他还吸取了一些少数民族医学的疗法，如治疗伤寒阴证的蒙医秘方健阳丹（回春丹）等。其内容丰富，见解独到，为后世外治学的发展开辟了广阔的道路，影响深远，值得现代医学应用并深入研究。

吴尚先不拘于古、不拘于外、善于借鉴学习，是一位富有开拓精神的医学家。因其对中医外治法做出的杰出贡献，被后人誉为"外治宗师"。

## 十二、孟河丁氏与近代中医教育

孟河医派发源于 1626 年，是我国目前保存最完好、各科齐全、嫡传后学后嗣人数最多的中医门户之一，孟河医派以费、马、巢、丁四大家闻名，丁氏的代表正是丁甘仁先生，成名虽晚却可谓孟河医派集大成者。

丁甘仁，名泽周，常州孟河镇人。孟河镇名医辈出，而以马培之、费伯雄、巢崇山最为著名。丁家三世业医，堂兄丁松溪学医于孟河医派的奠基人费伯雄，尽得其传。丁甘仁自幼体弱多病，与中医汤药结下不解之缘，在孟河家乡起初受教于丁松溪，继而学医于圩塘马绍成，习外科于巢崇山，后又拜安徽伤寒名家汪莲石为师。晚年又钻研金元四医家及吴又可、叶天士、王孟英等学说，博采众长，融诸家之学于一身。临诊推崇张仲景，辨病审症求因，用药灵活施治，内外参合，表里并兼，自成一派。

清末民初，以孟河医派丁甘仁先生为代表的一批有志之士客观分析中、西医优势，主张中西医结合和中医现代化，树起捍卫振兴民族医药文化的大旗。丁先生以发扬中医为己任，立志兴学，培养后继人才，联合同道夏应堂、谢观等集资办学。1916 年，其创造性地将中国几千年中医师承及西方院校教育模式结合起来，创办了"上海中医专门学校"（现为上海中医药大学），于 1917 年 7 月正式开学，开创了近代中医教育的先河。接着先后成立沪南、沪北两所广益中医院，为在校学生提供临证实习基地。两年后，又创办了"女子中医专门学校"。他所著述的《脉学辑要》《医经辑要》《药性辑要》，均为早年上海中医专门学校课本。该校设置了生理解剖学、病理学等西医重点课程，吸收西医学知识为我所用，并组织学生到沪南、沪北广益中医院，临证学习，使理论与实践紧密结合，由此造就了大批高水平的中医人才。中华人民共和国成立后担任上海中医学院院长的程门雪、黄文东，以及著名中医丁济万、曹仲衡、刘佐彤、王一仁、盛梦仙、张伯臾、秦伯未等，均为早期毕业于上海中医专门学校的高材生。可谓"医誉满海上，桃李遍天下"。

丁甘仁先生创办了中国近代第一所中医学校，开创了近代中医教育的先河，改变了培养中医师承家传的单一方式，为推动近代中医药事业发展做出了巨大贡献。

## 十三、第一部综合性中医药词典——《中国医学大词典》

《中国医学大词典》是由谢观先生及其门人所编著的，成书于 1921 年。它是我国第一部综合性中医药词典，影响深远，至今仍是医史研究者案头必备的工具书。

谢观，字利恒，晚年自号澄斋老人，江苏武进人。其伯祖谢兰生、伯父谢葆初皆故里孟河镇名医，父谢钟英为地理学大家。因此谢观先生自幼遍览家藏地理图书，熟诵《黄帝内经》《难经》《伤寒论》《金匮要略》及本草经方等书。先生肄业苏州东吴大学，1905 年赴广东法政学院执教地理 3 年，回沪后任澄衷学堂校长。随后，先生曾先后两次入职上海商务印书馆。自清朝末年西医东渐，中西医之争一直未停，而当时的上海更是争论的中心战场。谢观先生认为，中医学博大精深，古今医籍汗牛充栋，或奥质而难明，或讹夺而莫正。故学医者多，通才者少，致使中医学遭人误解。因此，在谢观先生任上海神州中医大学校长时，在中医学界和商务印书馆要求下开始编纂《中国医学大词典》。先生带领 12 名门人，焚膏继晷，日夜辛勤，以历代学说制为条释，扩编成《中国医学大词典》。

《中国医学大词典》内容包括病名、药名、方名、身体、医家、医书、医学 7 大类，共 3.7 万余条目，约计 350 万字。排列方法以首字笔画为序，首字相同者则以次字笔画为序。为方便检索，还编有辞头索引、辞条索引。《中国医学大词典》包含两个鲜明的特点：第一，收书范围广，先生在序言中写道："网罗散佚，远逮三韩日本之书"；第二，收书量极大，先生在例言中云：《四库》著录之医籍，不过百余种，本书搜罗旧籍，傍及朝鲜人、日本人之著作，为提要两千余种，借为考订古今医籍之阶梯。"《中国医学大词典》于 1926 年 7 月修订再版，1933 年 8 月再次出版，并注明为"国难后第一版"。中华人民共和国成立后，商务印书馆为了配合中央政府贯彻落实党的中医政策，分别于 1954 年 12 月、1955 年 4 月与 8 月 3 次重印发行，使《中国医学大词典》遍布全国各地，甚至海外。毋庸讳言，《中国医学大词典》的注释也确实存在着一些错讹之处，若以现今通行辞书体例来衡量，也存在着一些不足，但瑕不掩瑜，它仍不失为嘉惠医林、启迪后学的重要工具书，在漫漫中医药历史长河中散发着熠熠光辉。

## 十四、中西医结合的先行者——张锡纯

张锡纯（1860—1933 年），字寿甫，祖籍山东诸城，河北省盐山县人，中西医汇通学派的代表人物之一，近现代中国中医学界的医学泰斗，被后世誉为"轩岐之功臣，医林之楷模"。1893 年张锡纯在第二次参加科举落第后，遵父命一边教书一边学习医学。1911 年张锡纯任军医正，开始了专业行医的生涯。1916 年，他在沈阳创办了我国第一个中医医院——立达中医院，并担任院长。他的著作《医学衷中参西录》，被称为"医家必读之书"。

衷中参西，优势互补。清末民初，西学东渐，张锡纯致力沟通中西医学，主张以中医为主体，取西医之长，补中医之短。他主张"欲求医学登峰造极，诚非沟通中西医不可"。他认为"兼采中西生理之学，更参以哲学家谈生理处，复以己意融会贯通之。生理既明，而养生之理寓其中矣；养生之理既明，而治病之理寓其中矣"。张锡纯从生理、病理、药理各方面积极寻找中医与西医的共通之处。通过比较，他得出结论"中西之论药性，凡其不同之处，深究之又皆可以相通也"。

倡导新说，精勤实践。张锡纯尊古而不泥古，敢于创新，不全于故纸中求学问。主张"读《内经》之法，但于其可信之处精研有得，即能开无限法门。其不可信之处，或为后世伪托，付之不论可也"。此外，张锡纯认为"天下事理之赜，非一一亲身经过，且时时留心，必不能确切言之"。为验证临证疗效，他曾嚼服甘遂一二钱，泻下大量水及凝痰，始悟其有开顽痰之功。嚼服花椒 30 粒，知其确有毒副作用。他将自己的临证心得反复印证，不断深化，自拟方子达 160 余首，被誉为"医学实验派大师"。

治学严谨，桃李天下。张锡纯的一生除了孜孜研究医学外，在 1928 年定居天津后，还创办国医函授学校，设立"中西汇通医社"，培养后继人才。及门弟子如隆昌周禹锡，如皋陈爱棠、李慰农，天津孙玉泉、李宝和，辽宁仲晓秋等均为一方名医。

张锡纯提出的"衷中参西"汇通原则，为现代中西医结合的先声。取西医之长为我所用，冲破前人承袭旧论，抛弃崇古之习气，接受实验科学思想，仍值得现在的每一位中医人借鉴、学习。

第六章

中医药的新生与辉煌

中华人民共和国成立以来，党和政府高度重视中医药事业发展，出台了一系列方针政策，始终坚持中西医并重，着力打造中医药和西医药相互补充、协调发展的中国特色医疗卫生服务体系和卫生健康发展模式。中医药在医疗、保健、科研、教育、产业、文化等方面均取得了丰硕成果。当前，中医药在国际传统医学领域的话语权和影响力持续提升，中医药已传播至196个国家和地区，成为中国与欧盟、非盟、拉共体以及上海合作组织、金砖国家等地区和组织合作的重要领域。凝聚着中华民族数千年智慧的中医药，正在新时代的历史坐标上扬帆起航，将为健康中国建设和人类健康事业做出更大的贡献。

## 一、毛泽东主席关心中医药

中华人民共和国成立之初，疫病丛生，缺医少药，医疗卫生条件非常落后，全国卫生形势非常严峻。当时全国西医仅有 2 万多人，中医虽有几十万人，但却不能正常发挥作用。面对这样的现状，毛泽东主席提出了一系列发展中医药的重要思想。1949 年，毛泽东主席在接见全国卫生行政人员代表时，从保护和发展中医药的角度着重指出，只有很好地团结中医，提高中医，搞好中医工作，才能担负起几亿人口艰巨的卫生工作任务。

毛泽东主席曾多次高度评价中医药的现实价值。他指出"中国医药是一个伟大的宝库，应当努力发掘，加以提高"，不仅从宏观上提出了一些促进中医药发展的措施，指明了中医药发展的路径，同时还对新中国中医药工作的实践进行具体的指导。在 20 世纪 50 年代，为了正确贯彻执行对待中医的方针政策，毛泽东主席几乎年年都要就中医药问题进行指导。他强调有条件的省市都要举办西医离职学习中医班，预期以两年为期。1954 年，毛泽东主席作出对中药及中医古籍问题的重要批示，指出中药应当很好地保护与发展，我国中药有几千年的历史，是祖国极宝贵的财富，如果任其衰落下去，那是我们的罪过。中医书籍应进行整理。应组织有学问的中医，有计划有重点地先将某些有用的，从古文译成现代文，时机成熟时应组织他们结合自己的经验编出一套系统的中医医书来。

新中国成立后一段时期内，中医药的发展遇到了一些迟滞与困难，存在轻视、歧视和排斥中医药的情况，如公费医疗制度不报销中药费用、大医院不吸纳中医师、中医进修学校鼓励中医改学西医、高等医学院校未设置中医药课程，甚至有文章公开声称中医是"封建

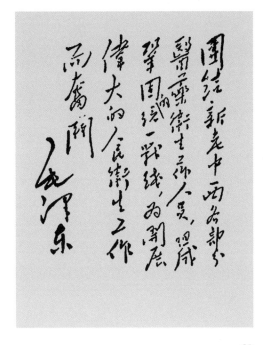

1950 年，毛泽东主席为第一届全国卫生工作会议题词："团结新老中西各部分医药卫生工作人员，组成巩固的统一战线，为开展伟大的人民卫生工作而奋斗！"

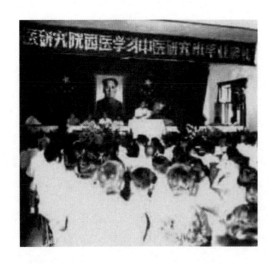

医"，鼓吹消灭中医。针对上述中医药发展过程中出现的问题，毛泽东主席提出了新中国卫生工作的3个基本原则"面向工农兵、预防为主、中西医结合"。这些思想和措施推动了中医药事业的发展和进步，为新中国中医药事业的蓬勃发展做出了重要贡献。

全国第一届西医学习中医学习班毕业典礼

## 二、用科学的方法研究中医——中医研究院成立

1950年，第一届全国卫生工作会议把团结中西医定为卫生工作的重要方针之一，彻底纠正了以往遗留下来的轻视、歧视、排斥中医的思想。在党和政府的关心支持下，中医药学进入了全新的发展阶段。1954年6月，毛泽东主席指示："即时成立中医研究机构，罗致好的中医进行研究，派好的西医学习中医，共同参加研究工作。"1954年10月26日，政务院文化教育委员会党组向中央提出了《关于改进中医工作问题的报告》，在报告中建议"成立中医研究院"，中央随后迅速批示"批准执行"。从1954年10月到1955年12月，经过一年多紧锣密鼓的筹建，接收了卫生部针灸疗法实验所等多家单位，基本完成中医研究院建设的筹备工作。

1955年12月19日，中华人民共和国卫生部中医研究院成立大会在北京市广安门内北线阁院部礼堂隆重举行。周恩来总理为中医研究院建院亲笔题词："发扬祖国医药遗产，为社会主义建设服务。"卫生部任命鲁之俊为首任中医研究院院长，朱琏、田润芝为副院长，彭泽民为名誉院长，萧龙友为名誉副院长。当天，到会祝贺的有李济深、谢觉哉、习仲勋、徐特立、张际春等领导。全国政协、统战部、国务院、卫生部等有关部门人员约400人应邀出席。

中医研究院成立之后，从全国各地选调30余位著名中医药专家，建立了8个机构，开展内、外、妇、儿、骨伤、眼科以及针灸、中药等方面的科研、临床和教育工作，为中医事业的发展培养了大批高级人才，使中医药成为我国防治疾病力量的重要组成部分，开启了用科学方法研究中医药的新时代。

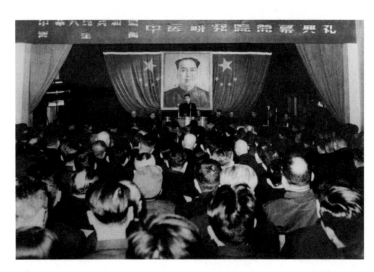

中华人民共和国卫生部
中医研究院成立大会
会场（1955年）

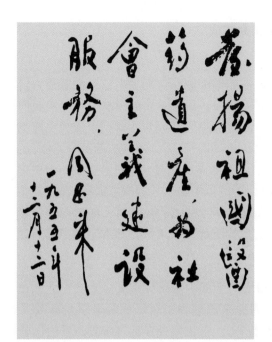

中医研究院的成立，标志着学习、整理和提高中医学遗产的工作，开始在专门机构的统一指导下科学地、有组织地进行。经过几代人的努力，中医研究院于 2005 年更名为中国中医科学院，发展成为一所集科研、医疗、教育、产业于一体的国家级综合性中医药科研机构，引领着全国中医药事业不断向前发展。

1955 年，周恩来总理为中医研究院建院时题词

### 三、中医药工作进入自立发展新时期——国家中医管理局成立

国家中医管理局诞生前，我国并没有独立的中医药管理机构，中医药工作一直由原卫生部中医司管理，中医药工作在我国的医疗卫生事业中一直处于从属地位。1978 年，中药工作从卫生部分出，归至国家医药管理局管理，中医、中药面临着"分家"状态。面对中医药管理和发展中存在的严峻问题，中医界反应十分强烈。1984 年，何任、张灿玾、李今庸等 10 位全国著名的中医专家，呈书国务院，陈述制约中医药发展的严重制度缺陷，恳切希望建立独立的中医药管理系统，成立国家中医药管理局。曾经担任卫生部副部长兼第一任国家中医药管理局局长的胡熙明也提出，"要想将中医药发扬光大，就要实行中医药自主管理"。行业内外强烈的呼声引起了党中央的高度重视。

党中央、国务院 5 次讨论中医问题。经过深入的调查研究，1986 年 1 月 4 日，国务院第九十四次常务会议决定成立国家中医管理局。会议指出，"要把中医摆在一个重要的位置。中西医结合是正确的，但不能用西医改造中医。西医要发展，中医也要发展，不能把中医只当成西医的从属"。1986 年 7 月 20 日，国务院正式下达了《关于成立国家中医管理局的通知》，明确规定"国家中医管理局是国务院直属机构，由卫生部代管。其主要任务是管理中医事业和中医人才培养等工作，继承发扬中医药学，为建设具有中国特色的社会主义卫生事业、提高我国人民的健康水平服务"。

国家中医药管理局的成立，体现了党和政府对中医药事业发展的高度重视。从此之后，中医药工作由过去的从属地位时期进入自立发展的新时期。中医药事业发展政策和机制不断完善，中医药科研内涵建设不断加强，中医防治疾病能力不断提高，中医药事业呈现出蓬勃繁荣的新局面。

## 四、中医战 SARS 震惊世界

2003 年春天，一场突如其来的严重急性呼吸综合征（SARS）疫情悄然而至。这是人类在 21 世纪发现的首个烈性传染病，来势汹汹，令人措手不及。2003 年 2 月中下旬，SARS 疫情在广东局部地区流行，3 月上旬在华北地区传播和蔓延，4 月中下旬疫情持续发展，人民身体健康与生命安全受到极大威胁。

北京是当时 SARS 疫情的重灾区。据 2003 年 4 月 29 日的统计数据显示，北京市累计确诊 SARS 病例 1347 人，疑似病例 1358 人，死亡病例 66 人，疫情异常严峻。而与此同时，广州传来了令人振奋的好消息，在著名中医专家邓铁涛治疗 SARS 的理论指导下，广州中医药大学第一附属医院实现了收治患者零死亡、零后遗症、院内零感染的良好战绩；广东省中医院共收治 112 例患者，治愈率超过 90%。4 月 7 日世界卫生组织（WHO）至广东省中医院考察，对该院使用中西医结合的方法治疗 SARS 给予高度评价。4 月 11 日卫生部非典型肺炎领导小组发布关于《非典型肺炎中医药防治技术方案（试行）》的通知。通知明确指出："广东省防治非典型肺炎的实践表明，采取中西医结合的防治方法优于单纯的西医方法。"2003 年 5 月 8 日，时任国务院副总理兼卫生部部长吴仪与在京的知名中医药专家座谈，强调中医是抗击 SARS 的一支重要力量，要充分认识中医药的科学价值，积极利用中医药资源，发挥广大医务人员的作用，中西医结合，共同完成防治 SARS 的使命。此次会议后，中医药正式进入北京抗击 SARS 的主战场。自 5 月 11 日开始，北京采取措施保障确保所有 SARS 定点医院都有中医药参与，多数住院患者使用中西医结合治疗 SARS，效果明显，北京的疫情逐渐得到控制。6 月初，中医专家进驻小汤山医院，中西医结合治疗方

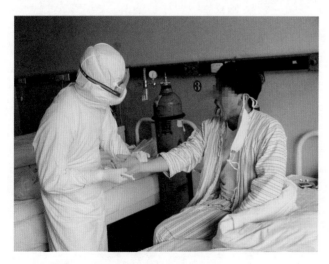

中医专家在北京地坛医院为 SARS 患者看舌诊脉

案得到了进一步的推广。6 月 24 日，WHO 宣布解除对北京的旅行警告，并将北京从"近期有当地传播"的 SARS 疫区名单中删除，标志着中国防治 SARS 工作取得了阶段性的重大胜利。

2003 年 10 月，WHO 和国家中医药管理局联合举办的中医、中西医结合治疗 SARS 国际研讨会在北京开幕，来自 WHO 的 17 名国际专家听取了中医药参与 SARS 防治的研究报告，与会专家一致认为，中西医结合治疗 SARS 是安全的，诸多方面具有潜在效益，高度评价了中西医结合方案在治疗 SARS 中发挥的重要作用。

## 五、首位获得诺贝尔生理学或医学奖的中国人——屠呦呦

2015 年 10 月 5 日，"诺贝尔生理学或医学奖"获奖名单揭晓，中国科学家屠呦呦因创新疟疾疗法的杰出贡献获奖。这是中国科学家因在本土进行科学研究而首次获得诺贝尔科学奖，也是我国医学界迄今为止获得的国际最高奖项。

屠呦呦，1930 年出生于浙江宁波。16 岁时，她曾因感染肺结核而被迫中止学业两年多，也是从那时起，正在读高中的屠呦呦便对医药学产生了浓厚的兴趣。1951 年，她考取北京医学院（现北京大学医学部）药学系，这个当时"冷门"的专业让她最终与中医药结缘。从北京医学院毕业后，屠呦呦一直在中医研究院（现中国中医科学院）工作。工作期间，她参加了卫生部全国第三期西医离职学习中医班的培训学习。

20 世纪 60 年代，氯喹抗疟失效，人类饱受疟疾之害。1969 年，中医研究院接受了国家疟疾防治项目"523"抗疟药研究任务。面对这个艰巨的任务，屠呦呦毅然扛起重担。她领导课题组从系统收集整理历代医籍、本草、民间方药入手，在收集 2000 余方药基础上，编写了 640 种药物为主的《抗疟单验方集》，并对其中的 200 多种中药开展实验研究，历经数百次实验，最终，以东晋医书《肘后备急方》"治寒热诸疟方"中提到的"青蒿一握。以水二升渍，绞取汁。尽服之"为参考，课题组利用现代医学和方法进行分析研究、不断改进提取方法，研究发现青蒿乙醚粗提取物的中性部分对疟原虫的抑制作用能达到 100%。经过进一步分离，1971 年，最终得到了对治疗疟疾有效的抗疟单体物质，也就是青蒿素。自青蒿素问世以来，已在全世界挽救了数百万人的生命。2021 年 6 月 30 日，世界卫生组织宣布中国获得无疟疾认证，中国疟疾感染病例由 20 世纪 40 年代的 3000 万减少至零，这是一个了不起的成就，青蒿素功不可没。

正如屠呦呦所说，青蒿素是传统中医药送给世界人民的礼物。几十年来，她和她的团队从未停下探索的脚步，她在中国传统医学与现代医学之间架起了一座桥梁，也为所有的科研人员打开了一扇走向世界的大门。

## 六、中国第一部中医药法颁布

2016 年 12 月 25 日，十二届全国人大常委会第二十五次会议表决通过《中华人民共和国中医药法》（以下简称《中医药法》），这标志着我国首部为传统中医药振兴而制定的国家法律的诞生。

早在 1983 年，全国人大代表董建华就提出了制定中医药法的议案，此后的历届全国人大及全国政协会上，不断有代表提出有关中医药立法的议案、提案。1986 年，时任国务院总理李鹏批示，先起草一部中医药振兴条例，待条件成熟后再立法。随后，国务院启动《中华人民共和国中医药条例》（以下简称《中医药条例》）的起草工作，并于 2003 年 4 月颁布该条例。随着我国中医药事业的不断发展，行业内外期望在《中医药条例》的基础上制定中医药法的呼声越来越强。根据国务院法制办和卫生部领导关于启动中医药立法起草工作的建议，国家中医药管理局于 2005 年 3 月启动了中医药法的起草工作，历经多次修改，几易其稿，2006 年形成了《中华人民共和国中医药法（草拟稿）》。2008 年 10 月，《中医药法》被列入了十一届全国人大常委会 5 年立法规划。2008—2015 年期间，国家中医药管理局重新组织中医药法的起草工作，在全国设立了 8 个课题组，分南北 2 个大组开展工作。经过多轮调研和专家论证，形成了新的《中医药法（草拟稿）》，并在 2011 年年底交由卫生部上报至国务院。国务院法制办多次征求中央有关部门、地方政府及部分医疗机构、高校和专家意见，9 次赴北京、内蒙古、广东、贵州等地进行实地调研，多次向社会公开征求意见，对《中医药法（草案）》进行不断的修改和完善。最终，于 2016 年通过全国人大常委会审议，由习近平主席签署主席令正式颁布。

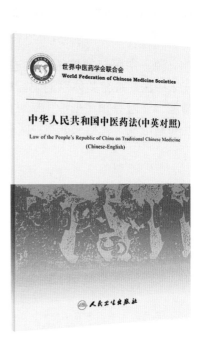

作为第一部全面、系统体现中医药特点的综合性法律，《中医药法》将党和国家关于发展中医药的方针政策用法律形式固定下来，将人民群众对中医药的期盼和要求用法律形式体现出来，体现了党和国家对中医药事业的高度重视，对中医药行业发展具有里程碑式的意义。

《中华人民共和国中医药法（中英对照）》，
人民卫生出版社 2017 年出版

## 七、传统医学正式进入《国际疾病分类第十一次修订本（ICD-11）》

2019 年 5 月 25 日，第 72 届世界卫生大会审议通过了《国际疾病分类第十一次修订本（ICD-11）》，首次纳入起源于中医药的传统医学章节，这是中国政府与中医专家历经十余年持续努力所取得的宝贵成果。

国际疾病分类（ICD）是世界卫生组织（WHO）制定颁布的、国际统一的疾病分类标准，是各国政府在医疗、管理、教学和科研及制定政策中关于疾病分类的规范性标准，也是全球卫生健康领域具有权威性的基础和通用标准之一。2007 年 WHO 启动 ICD 第 11 次修订工作后，国家中医药管理局组织了全国中医药系统专家进行研讨论证。2009 年，受国家中医药管理局委托，上海市中医药发展办公室（现上海市中医药管理局）承担起项目管理职责。由张伯礼院士、上海中医药大学教授严世芸等领衔的项目审评专家团队 36 人，还有全国近百名专家组成了术语、信息、标准、分类等各技术小组。在 WHO 的牵头组织和技术指导下，经过长期努力，最终在中国联合相关国家求同存异、通力合作下，ICD-11 将有关传统医学的补充章节纳入第 26 章，对起源于古代中国且当前在中国、日本、韩国和其他国家普遍使用的传统医学病证进行了分类，并将这一章节命名为 "Supplementary Chapter Traditional Medicine Conditions—Module I"，包括 150 条传统医学疾病和 196 条证候（不含特指和非特指病证）条目。该章节将中医诊断按病名（disorders）和证型（patterns）分别编码，前者如黄疸病（jaundice disorder），代码为 SA01；后者包括气虚（qi deficiency pattern），代码为 SE90 等；而每种疾病可由其症状、病因、病程和结果或治疗反应来定义。

源于中医药的传统医学进入 ICD-11 后，可与 ICD 体系同步推广传播，形成了中医病证分类体系的国际标准化语言，促进了中医药在临床、科研、教育、管理、保险等领域形成国际共识，增强了中医药服务统计信息的完整性、科学性和通用性，有利于推动中医药国际医疗服务的发展。

## 八、传承精华　守正创新——全面推进中医药振兴发展

党的十八大以来，以习近平同志为核心的党中央把传承创新发展中医药作为新时代中国特色社会主义事业的重要内容和中华民族伟大复兴的大事。2016年，《中医药发展战略规划纲要（2016—2030年）》发布，中医药发展上升为国家战略。2017年，《中华人民共和国中医药法》的实施为中医药事业发展提供了法律保障。2019年10月，《中共中央 国务院关于促进中医药传承创新发展的意见》印发，国务院召开全国中医药大会，全社会对中医药的认识提升到前所未有的高度。2022年，《"十四五"中医药发展规划》印发，对中医药发展作出了全局性、战略性、保障性规划。党的二十大报告中提出"促进中医药传承创新发展"，更为新时代中医药高质量发展进一步指明了前进方向。

在国家战略引领下，中医药全面融入健康中国行动。中医药服务能力进一步提升，人才队伍建设进一步加强，传承工作持续推进，科技创新取得新的突破。中医药事业发展硕果累累，在实践中书写了一个又一个辉煌篇章。2019年，中医药领域第一批国家临床医学研究中心获批；同年，全球首个中医药领域的循证医学中心在中国中医科学院成立。2020年，第四次全国中药资源普查工作完成，调查获取了200多万条调查记录，汇总了1.3万余种中药资源的种类和分布等信息。2021年，由哈佛医学院马秋富教授团队与复旦大学王彦青教授、中国中医科学院针灸研究所景向红教授团队完成的"A neuroanatomical basis for electroacupuncture to drive the vagal—adrenal axis"（中文标题：《电针驱动迷走神经——肾上腺轴的神经解剖学基础》），在国际顶尖杂志 Nature 正刊发表。2022年，国家中医药管理局首次牵头制定中医药人才工作政策性文件《关于加强新时代中医药人才工作的意见》。2023年，历时11年，由全国28家单位、34个课题组近千人参与编纂的《中华医藏》首批图书在国家图书馆发布。

中医药学包含着中华民族几千年的健康养生理念及其实践经验，凝聚着中国人民和中华民族的博大智慧。惟有传承精华，才能让中医药发展源远流长；惟有守正创新，才能为中医药发展注入源源不断的活力。传承精华，守正创新，在新的历史起点上，中医药必将焕发无限生机，为健康中国建设提供强劲动力，为构建人类命运共同体发挥出更大作用。

# Historical Narratives
## of TCM

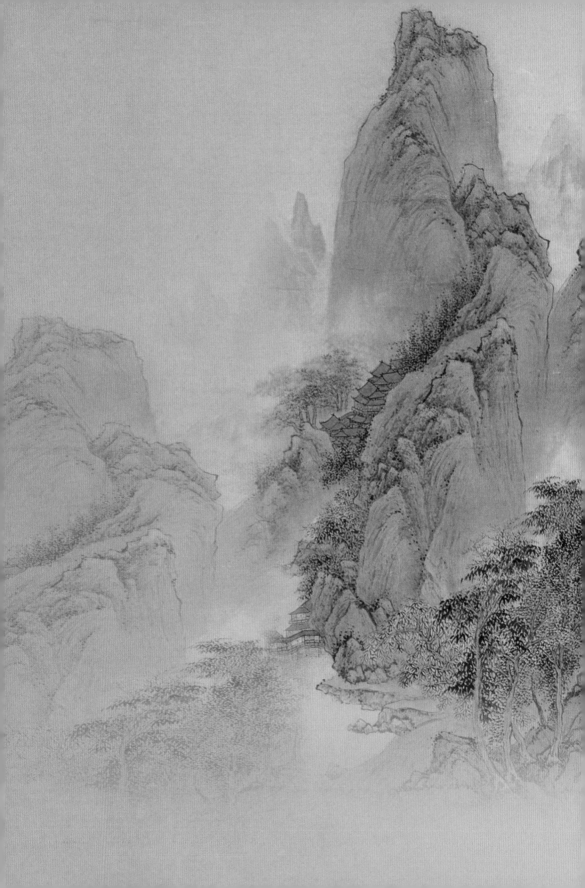

Chapter 1

Origin and Theoretical Formation

of Traditional Chinese Medicine

In Chinese history, there are many legends about the origin of traditional Chinese medicine (TCM). For thousands of years, some of these stories passed down from mouth to mouth in China have a strong mythic flavor. These stories and legends reflect the primitive medical and health knowledge accumulated by the ancient Chinese people in their daily life and production practices, seeking for survival, constantly exploring and summarizing their experience of fighting against diseases. In this long historical process, the earliest representative doctors and works of TCM theory were born, and these valuable experiences laid an important foundation for the establishment of the theoretical system of TCM later.

## I Shennong and All Kinds of Plants

Shennong is the legendary leader of Jiang tribe in ancient times. He lived in the Yellow River Basin 5,000 to 6,000 years ago. In ancient China, he was the Earth Emperor, one of the Three Emperors (Heaven Emperor, Earth Emperor, and Tai Emperor—Emperor of humans). Shennong invented slash-and-burn farming, created two kinds of earth-turning tools, taught tribal people to reclaim wasteland and plant crops, and made pottery and cooking utensils for diet. Therefore, Shennong was regarded as the founder of farming culture by later generations and was honored as "the first emperor of Five Grains" and "Shennong Emperor".

The legend that Shennong founded pharmacology by tasting all kinds of herbs has been passed down from ancient times. There is a record in *Huai-nan tzu– Management Instruction* that "Shennong tasted hundreds of herbs and recognized the sweetness and bitterness of water springs... At this time, 70 poisons were encountered in a day". *Historical Records* also said that "Shennong made wax sacrifices, whipped vegetation with ochre, tasted herbs, and then there was medicine". In ancient times, human beings were living in very harsh conditions. Shennong empathized with the people's diseases and personally tasted all kinds of herbs to observe plants' cold, warm, placid and hot properties and recorded them to treat the people. Legend has it that his body was transparent, and his internal organs were clearly visible so that he could see the conditions of the plants he ate in his body, so he could identify the varieties of plants that could cure diseases and save people. Shennong vowed to taste all kinds of herbs to relieve people's suffering. According to the legend, he once tasted 70 types of poisons in one day and was poisoned many times. Later, he died from a bitter taste of *Gelsemium elegans*. In order to commemorate Shennong's kindness and achievements, people worshiped him as the "God of Medicine". Objectively speaking, after the rise of primitive agriculture, people paid more attention to the properties of plants to find better types of crops. They needed to know whether the food was poisonous or edible, distinguish the tastes of different parts of plants and their efficacies. On this basis, the concept of medicine was gradually shaped and medical exploration began. It can be said that the concept of medicine was formed in the process of people's daily life, a kind of "an untended willow growth", which also roughly reflects the historical origin of Shennong's legend of tasting herbs.

Shennong's legendary stories of tasting herbs reflect the practical process of people's discovery and understanding of medicine, from which we can also speculate that the practical experience in labor, production, and life is the source of the development of TCM. The view that "medicine originates from sage" reflects the accumulation and contribution of different clans to medicine in the practice of fighting against diseases in ancient times. Shennong and Huangdi are the representatives of these clans, which also reflects people's respect for those who have made outstanding contributions in the development of medicine.

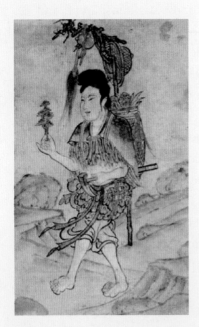

*Statue of Shennong*
(discovered in 1974 in the wooden tower of Fogong Temple in Mi County, Shanxi Province, painted in the Liao Dynasty)

Chapter 1   Origin and Theoretical Formation of Traditional Chinese Medicine

## II Fuxi and Bagua (Eight Trigrams)


Fuxi is one of the earliest Three Emperors recorded in China's ancient books and is the earliest documented creator in China. *The History of Three Sovereigns* records that Fuxi "has holy virtue while looking up at the sky and down at the earth". About the name Fuxi, there is no accurate record in history. Some people think that his surname is Fu, while others believe his surname is Feng (wind). The era in which Fuxi lived was the middle and late Neolithic Age, a brutal era. Fuxi invented the method of drilling wood for the fire, bringing people warmth and light and significantly improving their living conditions. The people admired and appreciated him so much that they made him emperor.

In ancient times, people were ignorant of nature phenomena, such as wind, and rain, lightning and thunder. People didn't know the reasons, and they were confused and afraid. To find out the causes of these natural phenomena, Fuxi looked up at the sky, looked down at the ground, and studied the footprints of birds and beasts and the textures of animals carefully. The *Book of History–The Book of Zhou–Gu Ming* pseudo-Kong Anguo said: "In the period of Fuxi King, he saw Longma (horse-like dragons, an image in ancient China) swimming in the river, so he drew the eight trigrams based on the pattern of the dragon." This passage records the story of Fuxi painting the Bagua (eight trigrams) while watching dragons and horses. In ancient times, in the tributary of the Yellow River in today's Luoyang, there appeared a sea beast which looked like a camel with left and right wings, horse body, dragon scales, and a height of eight chi and five cun. This sea beast walked in the rough waves and people called it Longma because it looked like a dragon and a horse. Longma carried a river map on its back, and the spots on it were regular and beautiful. Looking closely, they were left 38, right 49, middle 50, and rear 16. After hearing about it, Fu Xi came to watch it, and he drew the original Bagua (eight trigrams) with this inspiration at the Bagua Desk in Tianshui (Gansu Province). The Bagua (eight trigrams) are the earliest written symbols in China, which combine the principles of yin and yang and five elements, and are tools for deducing world space and time. Fuxi's Bagua, also called innate eight trigrams, were used by King Wen of the later Zhou Dynasty to deduce 64 hexagrams based on the Bagua (eight trigrams), which is known as the *Book of Changes* today. Huangfu Mi, the famous medical scientist and writer in the Western Jin Dynasty, recorded in *Emperor Century*: "Fuxi painted the Bagua (eight trigrams) ... the principles of all diseases can be classified." According to this, later generations inferred that Fuxi played a pioneering and vital role in the development of TCM.

The invention and spread of the Bagua (eight trigrams) made it easier for the ancients to travel long distances without being lost because they couldn't remember where they came from. They could solve the direction problem with the Bagua (eight trigrams) gnomon and a few brighter stars. To commemorate the great achievement of Fuxi in inventing the Bagua (eight trigrams), later generations called the Bagua (eight trigrams) "Fuxi Bagua" and they called the river haunted by Longma Tuhe ( 图河 ).

## III TCM in *The Book of Songs*

*The Book of Songs* is the earliest collection of poems in China, which was created from the early Western Zhou Dynasty to the middle of the Spring and Autumn Period. It has been sung in China for thousands of years and is a well-known classic of Chinese studies because of its beautiful rhythm, sincere emotion, and artistic conception. *The Book of Songs* reflects all aspects of people's social life from the Western Zhou Dynasty to the Spring and Autumn Period, such as farming, sericulture, picking, weaving, dyeing, construction, animal husbandry, etc. At the same time, it also records many contents related to medicine, which reflects the medical development level at that time to a certain extent.

Among the 305 articles in *The Book of Songs*, 144 are related to plants, and more than 50 plant species are recorded, including the collection seasons and producing areas of some plants. Although there are few descriptions of the direct use of drugs to treat diseases in the book, many records related to TCM and ancient people's lives are revealed between the lines of the poems. For example, *Ballad from Wei State–Bo Xi* wrote, "How can you get Xuancao ( 谖草 )? On the back of the tree." It's recorded in the poem that Xuancao ( 谖草 ) can relax emotions and make people forget their worries. Xuancao ( 谖草 ) is the Xuancao (*Hemerocallis fulva* L., 萱草 ) we call today. Another example is "Let's pick the brightly colored Fuyi ( 芣苢 )" written in *Ballad from Zhounan State–Fuyi*, a folk song sung by rural women who were collecting Fuyi ( 芣苢 ). Fuyi ( 芣苢 ) is Cheqiancao (*Plantago asiatica* L. or *Plantago depressa* Willd.). Both its herb and seed are for medicinal use. The property of Cheqianzi (Semen Plantaginis) is sweet, bland, and cold, which relieves stranguria by diuresis. From the Shang and Zhou Dynasties to the Han and Jin Dynasties, most doctors believed that Cheqianzi (Semen Plantaginis) had the effect of strengthening yin, nourishing essence, and contributing to fertility.

*The Book of Songs* also contains a simple view of health cultivation in TCM. In the primitive farming society, people depended on the grace of nature to a large extent for their clothing, food, shelter, and transportation. Therefore, the ancients were full of reverence for nature and gradually accumulated rich experience in adapting to nature in their daily life. The idea of "harmony man and nature" and "adapting to nature" was reflected in *The Book of Songs*. For example, *Ballad from Bin State–July* records, "In July, the fire falls to the west, and in September, women sew clothes to protect against cold ... In April, Yuanzhi blossoms, and in May, the robin cries out; in August, the fields are busy with the harvest; in October, the leaves fall from the trees..." According to the order of 12 months a year, it introduces the daily life and work of the ancients in accordance with the season, showing the picture of harmonious coexistence between man and nature. There are also aesthetics and pursuits of the ancients in diet in the book. For example, *Eulogy of Shang Dynasty–Ancestors* records that "The diet should be abstinent and moderate", reflecting the ancient people's view of diet and health that harmony is beauty, which has a far-reaching influence on the health cultivation theory of later generations.

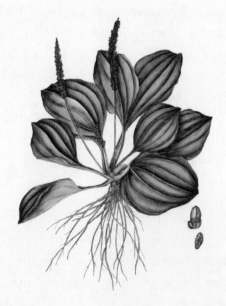

*Cheqiancao*
(Herba Plantaginis)

## IV The Cornerstone of TCM Theory—*Huangdi's Cannan of Inner Classic*

*Huangdi's Cannan of Inner Classic* (most commonly known as *Huangdi Neijing, Neijing* for short) is the earliest existing medical work with a relatively complete theory in China, and it is also one of the four classic works of TCM. Huangdi, named Xuanyuan, is the first of the Five Emperors in *Historical Records* and is a mythical figure in ancient times. He unified the Central Plains, taught the people to sow grain, developed Chinese characters, made heavenly stems and earthly branches and musical instruments, and was the forefather of the Chinese nation. Although *Huangdi Neijing* is named after Huangdi, it may not have been written by him. Because Huangdi is the first ancestor of China and has had a significant influence on the development of Chinese civilization, scholars later used the name Huangdi to improve the authoritativeness of their works. Most modern scholars believe that *Huangdi Neijing* was not written by one person, but the experience and theoretical summary of many dynasties and doctors.

*Huangdi Neijing* was first published in the *Book of Han–Record of Art and Culture*, including *Plain Questions* and *Miraculous Pivot*. The original book has 9 volumes, 9 chapters in each volume, 81 chapters in total, totaling 18 volumes with 162 chapters, covering human physiology, anatomy, pathology, diagnosis, treatment principles, disease prevention, etc. *Plain Questions* focuses on the fundamental theories of human physiology and pathology and disease treatment in TCM, while *Miraculous Pivot* stresses on acupuncture and moxibustion theory, and collaterals theory, and human anatomy. *Huangdi Neijing* has had a great influence on later generations, and is still a symbol of Chinese culture to this day. Its main achievements are divided into three aspects: firstly, it introduces the theory of correspondence between man and universe, yin and yang and five elements. From the wholeness of human body itself and the unity of man and nature, the holistic view of TCM is explained systematically and completely. Secondly, the concepts of anatomy and blood circulation are discussed. Thirdly, it emphasizes the idea of disease prevention in early treatment. The idea of "treating the disease before it arises" in TCM comes from *Huangdi Neijing*.

*Huangdi Neijing* is a comprehensive summary of TCM theories from the times of Fuxi, Shennong, and Huangdi to the Qin and Han Dynasties. It is the earliest existing classical medical masterpiece that comprehensively and systematically expounds the theoretical system of TCM in China. It marks the rise of TCM from experience accumulation to the stage of theoretical summary and the completion of the initial construction of TCM theoretical system. Until today, it still effectively guides the theoretical development and clinical practice of TCM. As a classic of Chinese traditional culture, *Huangdi Neijing is* not only a medical masterpiece but also a profound cultural masterpiece. With life as the center, this book discusses the interrelation among heaven, earth, and man, and analyzes the most basic proposition of medical scienc—the law of life and establishes the corresponding theoretical system and the principles and techniques of disease prevention and treatment. It contains the rich knowledge of philosophy, politics, astronomy, and other disciplines and is an encyclopedia about life.

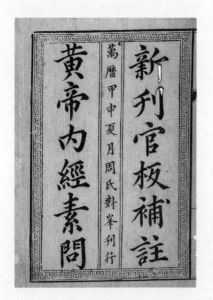

*Photoprint of Huangdi's Cannon of Inner Classic*
*Plain Questions*
(Huáng Dì Nèi Jīng Sù Wèn, 黄帝内经素问 )
now preserved in the Library of China Academy
of Chinese Medical Sciences (CACMS)

# V The First Pharmacology Monograph—*Shennong's Classic of Materia Medica*

*Shennong's Classic of Materia Medica*, referred to as *Herbal Classic* or *Materia Medica Classic*, is the first systematic summary of Chinese pharmacology. It's also one of the four classic works on TCM and the earliest known work of Chinese materia medica. There are different opinions about the time when it was written. It is said that it originated from Shennong, and most medical historians think that it was written in the Eastern Han Dynasty. Just as *Huangdi Neijing* is named after Huangdi, this book is entitled *Shennong's Classic of Materia Medica*, because, for one thing, there is a legend that Shennong tasted hundreds of herbs and discovered medicines since ancient times, for another, it is a response of respect for antiquity.

*Shennong's Classic of Materia Medica* is the first systematic summary of TCM in China and it is divided into three volumes, containing 365 kinds of medicinals, which are classified into top grade, middle grade and low grade according to the tripartite classification. *Shennong's Classic of Materia Medica—Prologue* compiled by Sen Lizhi recorded, "A total of 120 kinds of top grade medicinals belongs to the sovereign drug, which dominate the nourishment of life to adapt to the Heaven, and is non-toxic. It will not hurt him if one takes it more or for a long time. It also relaxes him, benefits his qi, keep him young and prolong his life. A total of 120 kinds of middle grade medicinals belongs to minister drug, which cultivates one's nature to adapt to him, and is non-toxic or toxic. To cure a disease and replenish deficiency, this category is a good choice. A total of 125 kinds of low grade medicinals belongs to the assistant drug, which is mainly used to treat diseases to adapt to Earth. Most of them are toxic and must not be taken for a long time. To eliminate cold-heat pathogens, unblock the accumulation and cure the disease, this category is a good choice."

Most of the theories and compatibility rules of Chinese materia medica in *Shennong's Classic of Materia Medica* and the principle of harmony of seven emotions have played a significant role in medication practice for thousands of years and are the sources of the development of TCM pharmacology theory. Based on the analysis of the description of various drugs in the book, it mainly covers the most common used names of medicinals, other names of medicinals, places of production, growing environment, harvesting, storage, processing, identification, quality identification, classification, property, flavor, efficacy, indications, contraindications, usage, the law of compatibility and application of medicinals, the sovereign (chief), minister (associate), adjuvant (assistant) and courier (guide) of formulas and the principles of composition, which basically construct the theoretical framework of Chinese materia medica. Its advent marks the initial construction and formation of the theoretical system of Chinese materia medica. The theories and principles of medicinal property and flavor, efficacy, indications, and clinical use recorded in the book have been effectively guiding the clinical practice of TCM and playing a positive role in the medical care of people in later generations. However, due to the limitations of the historical conditions at that time, there were also some mistakes in *Shennong's Classic of Materia Medica*. The theology of divination in the Eastern Han Dynasty and the Taoist pursuit of "immortal way" directly or indirectly influenced the book. For example, it was recorded that "Xionghuang (Realgar)... is refined and eaten to make immortals lighter", and "mercury... is taken for a long time, and immortals never die", which had a negative impact on the development of pharmacology in later generations.

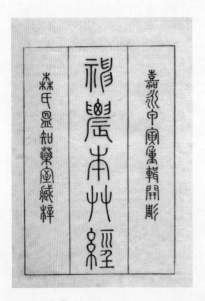

*Photoprint of Shennong's Classic of Materia*
(Shén Nóng Běn Cǎo Jīng, 神农本草经 )
now preserved in the Library of CACMS

# VI The Guiding Work of TCM Theory—*Classic of Questioning*

*Eighty-one Classic of Questioning of Yellow Emperor*, referred to as *Classic of Questioning* (Nàn Jīng, 难经) or *Eighty-one* Questioning for short, is another theoretical work of TCM following *Huangdi Neijing*. There are two interpretations of the word "nàn" in the book's title: first, the content is esoteric and difficult to understand. For example, *Reading Records of County* written by Chao Gongwu in the Southern Song Dynasty recorded: "According to the essence of *Huangdi Neijing*, eighty-one chapters are far-reaching and not easy to understand. Hence it was called *Classic of Questioning*." Second, it is asking difficult questions, that is, *The Emperor's Time in China* written by Huangfu Mi recorded: "*Huangdi Neijing* is to ask eighty-one questions." "Jīng" refers to *Huangdi Neijing*. Although *the Classic of Questioning* and *Huangdi Neijing* are not necessarily related to the inheritance of medical knowledge, they build the foundation of the TCM theoretical system and play a crucial role in the formation and development of TCM theory.

*The Classic of Questioning* mainly explains and gives play to the gist of *Huangdi Neijing*. Its content and style are compiled in a hypothetical way of asking & answering questions and explaining difficulties, and it discusses 81 medical theories. The contents are brief and concise with detailed analysis, involving human physiology, pathology, diagnosis and treatment of diseases, among which the discussion on acupuncture and moxibustion is particularly highlighted, and 32 of the 81 difficulties are involved in them.

*The Classic of Questioning* not only analyzes the gist of *Huangdi Neijing* but also gives a pioneering play to the theories of TCM. It can be said that it supplements what *Huangdi Neijing* has not discussed, expanding the ideas of the former saints and enlightening the counterparts of the later generation, which has had a far-reaching impact on the development of TCM theory in the later generation. The book records the pulse diagnosis method of "taking Cunkou alone", the triple energizer and vital gate theory, and the therapy of reinforcing and reducing manipulations of acupuncture, which were revered by doctors of all ages. When Wang Shuhe wrote *Pulse Classic* in Wei and Jin Dynasties, he inherited the pulse diagnosis method of *Classic of Questioning*. In addition, channel & collateral theory, acupoint function, and acupuncture operation were given more play in the *Classic of Questioning*, which also had a very important influence on the formation and development of acupuncture and moxibustion in TCM. Therefore, many doctors in the past dynasties attached importance to the *Classic of Questioning* and gave it a higher evaluation. In the Qing Dynasty, *Preface of Annotation to Classic of Questioning* written by Xu Lingtai, once commented: "Only the *Classic of Questioning* is to understand the content of the *Huangdi Neijing*, to spread its essence, and people regard this book as the most authoritative annotation." Since the Eastern Han Dynasty, as one of the classic works of traditional Chinese medicine, *Classic of Questioning* is a classic work used by ancient Chinese medical scientists to explore the medical theory, state their opinions and distinguish right from wrong.

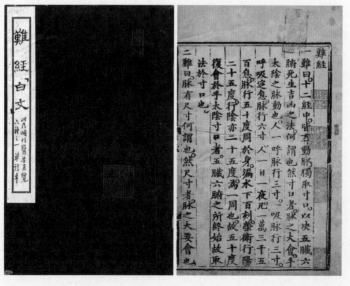

*Photoprint of Classic of Questioning* (Nàn Jīng, 难经) now preserved in the Library of CACMS

Chapter 2

Qin, Han, Jin, Southern and Northern Dynasties

—TCM Clinical Practice and Academic Collation

The development of medicine is closely related to many factors, such as social politics, economy, and culture at that time. From Qin and Han Dynasties to Jin and Southern and Northern Dynasties in Chinese history, there were both the feudal dynasties with a high concentration of imperial power and the period of vassal separatism with frequent wars and social unrest. Correspondingly, the development of TCM experienced a period of overall improvement and a short period of stagnation. Generally speaking, the medical experience of TCM was continuously accumulated and enriched after hundreds of years of development, the clinical field was continuously expanded, the theory of TCM was tested more in practice, and the medical system was further improved and enriched, which laid a solid foundation for the significant development of TCM in the Sui and Tang Dynasties.

## I The Magic Doctor Bian Que

Bian Que was the most influential medical scientist in China during the pre-Qin period and the first medical scientist with a formal biography in Chinese medical history. His life story was published in Sima Qian's *Historical Records–Biography of Bian Que and Canggong*. Bian Que, with Qin as his last name, Yueren as his first name, born in the 5th century BC, was a famous doctor in Warring States Period. According to legend, people called a magic doctor Bian Que in the ancient Xuanyuan era. As a result of his excellent medical skills and miraculous curative effects in treating diseases, people associated him with Bian Que, an ancient highly-skilled doctor, and later simply called him "Bian Que".

Bian Que was well versed in four examinations: inspection, auscultation and olfaction, inquiry and palpation, and especially in inspection and pulse-taking. According to the records of *Historical Records–Biography of Bian Que and Canggong*, Bian Que judged the illness and approximate time of death of Lord of Qi State only through observation. This was the source of Zhang Zhongjing's "looking at the color of Lord of Qi" in the preface to *Treatise on Febrile Diseases*, which reflected Bian Que's superb observation level and also showed that he attached great importance to disease prevention. He repeatedly persuaded Lord of Qi to treat as soon as possible, indicating he had the idea of preventing diseases before they happened. At the same time, Bian Que was also very proficient in pulse theory, especially famous for pulse-taking. It is recorded in *Historical Records* that once, Zhao Jianzi, a leader of Zhao State, suddenly fell ill and became unconscious for five days. The officials of Zhao State were very panic. After taking Zhao Jianzi's pulse, Bian Que thought that the patient's blood flow was normal without any death syndrome. After treatment, Zhao Jianzi recovered as expected. This incident fully demonstrates Bian Que's superb pulse-taking diagnosis technique. Sima Qian praised him: "Up to now, Bian Que is the best doctor of the pulse diagnosis in the world."

Bian Que not only had superb medical skills but also always adhered to the medical principle of "six untreatable", which is recorded in *Historical Records–Biography of Bian Que and Canggong*, "The first untreatable condition is arrogance and unreasonableness; the second untreatable condition is despising health but valuing money; the third untreatable condition is inappropriate clothing and diet; the fourth untreatable condition is disharmony of yin and yang, and dysfunction of zang-fu viscera; the fifth untreatable condition is a weak body that cannot withstand the power of medicine; the sixth untreatable condition is belief in witchcraft but not in medicine." The principle of "six untreatable" symbolizes Bian Que's noble medical ethics and materialism against superstitious witchcraft.

Most of the stories about Bian Que are collected from the folk community, and passed down from mouth to mouth, so, misinformation is inevitable. However, because of his important contribution to the development of TCM, people have highly respected Bian Que since Qin and Han Dynasties, and temples and tombs have been built for him in various places to commemorate this outstanding folk doctor and outstanding medical scientist.

## II Chunyu Yi and Ancient Medical Records

Chunyu Yi is the only medical scientist recorded in the official history of the Western Han Dynasty. Chunyu Yi (about 215–150 BC), surnamed Chunyu, named Yi, was born in Linzi, and used to be the "Taicang Chief" of Qi, so people also called him "Taicang Gong" or "Canggong". According to *Historical Records–Biography of Bian Que and Canggong*, Chunyu Yi loved medicine since childhood and once took many famous doctors as teachers. Sima Qian appraised him like this, "He treats people and judges whether they live or die, and his judgement is borne out in most cases."

In the fourth year of Emperor Wen of the Han Dynasty, Chunyu Yi was falsely accused, arrested, and imprisoned. His youngest daughter, Ti Ying, petitioned to Emperor to save her father. Emperor Wen of Han was moved by her filial piety and released Chunyu Yi. This is the story of "Ti Ying saving her father" in history. Later, Emperor Wen summoned him and asked him many questions, such as studying medicine, diagnosing and treating diseases, and taking apprenticeship, etc. Chunyu Yi answered them one by one. He introduced in detail the name, gender, residence, occupation, disease, treatment, therapeutic effect, prognosis and other information of 25 patients treated, which was called "diagnosis records" at that time. Later, Sima Qian recorded these 25 medical cases in *Historical Records–Biography of Bian Que and Canggong*, which became the earliest existing medical cases recorded in Chinese literature.

"Medical cases" objectively reflect Chunyu Yi's medical thoughts and characteristics of diagnosis and treatment. In terms of understanding the etiology, Chunyu Yi thinks it includes the following factors: natural factors (wind, cold, summer-heat, heat, flooding, etc.), improper diet, emotional overreaction, overwork and unhealthy way of life. For example, obesity can be caused by little activity, and dental caries may result from "the invasion of wind pathogen, sleeping with mouth open and non-rinsing of the mouth after eating". Among the 25 medical cases recorded, 20 cases had pulse manifestation, and ten of them were judged solely by pulse manifestation. Statistically, there are nearly 20 kinds of pulse manifestations in the book, such as floating, deep, stringy, tight, rapid, slippery, choppy, long, large, intermittent, weak, and scattered. Except for normal, drum, static, and manic pulse, which have not been used in later generations, other pulse manifestations are still in use today. In treating diseases, Chunyu Yi mainly uses drugs, acupuncture, moxibustion, and other methods, some of which are used alone and some in combination. These diagnoses and treatment methods have contributed to the development of TCM theory and clinical medicine.

Chunyu Yi's "medical cases" not only preserved the relevant materials in the medical literature before the Western Han Dynasty but also reflected the actual level of TCM in the early Western Han Dynasty. Moreover, it truthfully recorded his experience in treating diseases, which has a very high research value in the medical history of our country and played a positive role in promoting the development of TCM.

## III The Originator of Surgery Hua Tuo and Powder for Anesthesia

Hua Tuo, named Yuanhua, a native of Qiao County in Pei (now Bozhou, Anhui Province), was a famous medical scientist in the late Eastern Han Dynasty in China. Hua Tuo, Dong Feng and Zhang Zhongjing were called "Jian'an Three Imperial Doctors". Hua Tuo was familiar with all kinds of medical books and was good at internal and external medicine, gynecology, pediatrics, acupuncture and moxibustion, etc. The methods of his treatment were varied, and his prescriptions were sophisticated. Besides, his medical practice covered parts of Jiangsu, Shandong, Henan, and Anhui provinces. He cured countless patients and was deeply loved and respected by the general public.

Hua Tuo was famous for his medical skills all over the world. He once treated many influential figures in the Three Kingdoms Period. He gave Guan Yu "bone scraping treatment", treated incised wounds for Zhou Tai, a famous general of Wu Kingdom and treated internal injuries for Chen Deng, the prefecture chief of Guangling. Cao Cao, the prime minister at that time, suffered from intermittent headaches, which failed to be treated repeatedly. When he heard that Hua Tuo had superb medical skills, he asked Hua Tuo to treat him. After Hua Tuo gave him acupuncture treatment, it took effect quickly. Cao Cao was thrilled and forced Hua Tuo to be his doctor. However, Hua Tuo was indifferent to fame and wealth and didn't want his medical skills to be used only by the bigwigs, so he went home under the pretext and postponed his return. His behavior angered Cao Cao, which led him to be eventually killed by Cao Cao. Doctors of later generations all felt sorry for his death.

According to the historical records, Hua Tuo wrote various medical books, including *The Methods of Using Acupuncture and Moxibustion*, but unfortunately, they were all lost. Hua Tuo was the first doctor to perform surgery on patients in Chinese history. Hua Tuo's outstanding achievements in surgery were mainly in creating "Mafei" (powder for anesthesia) with wine and performing abdominal tumor resection, gastrointestinal anastomosis under general anesthesia. In the *History of the Late Han Dynasty–Biography of Hua Tuo*, it recorded, "If the disease is in the abdominal cavity and cannot be treated with acupuncture or medicine, the patient is ordered to take powder for anesthesia with wine first. When the patient gets unconscious, his abdomen is cut open and the mass is removed. If the disease is in the stomach, the stomach will be cut to rinse to get rid of the filth, and then sewed up. A magical ointment is applied to the wound, and the wound heals in four or five days. The patient returns to normal in a month." This passage tells future generations exactly that powder for anesthesia was taken with wine, and Hua Tuo skillfully used it to perform abdominal tumor resection, gastrointestinal resection and anastomosis, which significantly improved the operation efficiency and reduced the pain of patients. The general anesthesia surgery developed by Hua Tuo is unprecedented in the Chinese medical history and rare in the world medical history. Its invention and application are nothing short of remarkable in the medical history of the world, so Hua Tuo is also honored as the "originator of surgery" by later generations. People of all ages in China revere Hua Tuo so that his memorials are all over the country, such as "Hua's Ancestral Temple" in Bozhou, Anhui Province, "Hua Tuo's Temple" in Huazhuang, Xuzhou, and Hua Tuo's Tomb in Xuchang, Henan Province.

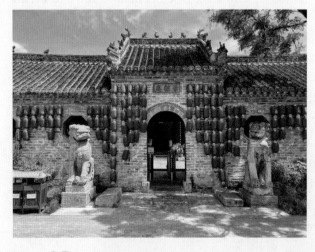

*Hua's Ancestral Temple*
Located in Bozhou City, Anhui Province

## IV The Medical Saint Zhang Zhongjing and *Treatise on Cold Pathogenic and Miscellaneous Diseases*

Zhang Zhongjing, a native of Nieyang, Nanyang County (now Dengzhou, Henan Province), was very talented and intelligent, especially interested in medicine when he was young. He was once taught by Zhang Bozu, a doctor in the same county. After years of hard work and clinical practice, his medical skills far exceeded his teacher's. Later generations honored him as a "Medical Saint" because of his outstanding contribution to TCM.

Zhang Zhongjing lived in the late Eastern Han Dynasty when the court was highly corrupt, eunuchs were in power, years of disasters and epidemics displaced people. Many doctors lost their medical ethics, resulting in many patients losing their lives. For example, "when they diagnose the pulse, they only press the cun pulse without touching the chi pulse, and they only press the hand pulse but not the foot pulse"; "when they diagnose a patient, they examine the patient for a while and then prescribe medicine". In such a situation, Zhang Zhongjing assiduously studied medical theoretical literature and referred to prescription works. He also extensively absorbed the clinical essence of the Han Dynasty and before it, and combined it with his long-term accumulated medical experience to compose *Treatise on Cold Pathogenic and Miscellaneous Diseases*. The original book, consisting of 16 volumes, was soon lost due to the war. The commonly used version nowadays is compiled by Wang Shuhe, and revised by medical officials Sun Qi, Lin Yi et al. during the Northern Song Dynasty, which was divided into *Treatise on Cold Pathogenic Disease* and *Synopsis of Golden Chamber*. *Treatise on Cold Pathogenic Disease* provides a comprehensive overview of the differentiation of syndromes and the rules of prescribing formulas for exogenous febrile diseases, while *Synopsis of Golden Chamber* mainly expounds on internal miscellaneous diseases. The two books are together called the Song version *Treatise on Cold Pathogenic and Miscellaneous Diseases* by later generations.

*Treatise on Cold Pathogenic and Miscellaneous Diseases*, which closely combined the basic theory of TCM with clinical practice, is also one of the most influential works in the history of TCM development. It took the holistic

99

concept as the guiding ideology, treating typhoid fever with six channels and miscellaneous diseases with zang-fu viscera and meridians; it is the first medical classic with principle, method, prescription, and medicine in China. TCM doctors in later generations paid much attention to study and research on it. After the Ming and Qing Dynasties, the study of *Treatise on Cold Pathogenic Diseases* became an academic school that has had an important impact to this day.

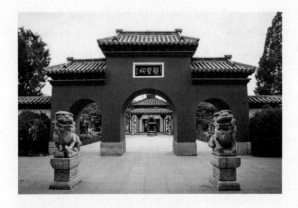

*The memorial temple of Zhang Zhongjing* located in Nanyang City, Henan Province

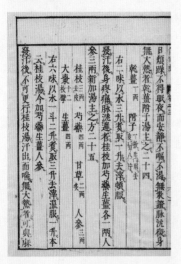

*Photoprint of Treatise on Cold Pathogenic Disease* (Shāng Hán Lùn，伤寒论) now preserved in the Library of CACMS

# V A Taoist and Medical Scientist—Ge Hong

Ge Hong (about 283–363 AD), Courtesy-named Zhichuan, and art-named Bao Pu Zi, was a famous Taoist theorist, medical scientist, and alchemist in Jin Dynasty. Born in an official family in Jurong, Danyang County (now Jurong County, Jiangsu Province), he wrote many books all his life, but most of them were lost. He once compiled 100 volumes of the large-scale medical book *Golden Chamber Prescription*, which were lost, and its contents are not known in detail. Considering that this book was so numerous that it was difficult to carry and retrieve, Ge Hong condensed the contents of common clinical diseases and emergencies into *Handbook of Rescue Prescription*, also known as *Handbook of Prescriptions for Emergency*, or *Handbook of Prescriptions* for short. The name of "handbook" means carrying it with you in case of emergency. As it's made for emergencies, the prescriptions in the book are classic and simple, and most of the medicines recorded are readily available and cheap, especially suitable for ordinary people's daily treatment and first aid. *Handbook of Prescriptions for Emergency* is one of the critical medical classics in the Jin and Southern and Northern Dynasties. Although there are not many volumes, the contents are rich and it is also the earliest existing monograph on emergency diagnosis and treatment.

*Handbook of Prescriptions for Emergency* is a comprehensive prescription book focusing on treating emergency diseases, which highlights the characteristics of simplicity, convenience, cheapness, and verification. The book records the treatment methods for tsutsugamushi disease, smallpox, rabies, and other diseases. In addition, the emergency treatment techniques created by Ge Hong contributed a lot to the clinical emergency treatment and greatly improved the emergency treatment level in ancient China, including artificial respiration, gastric lavage, drowning rescue pouring water method, abdominal puncture drainage method, urethral catheterization, enema and so on. In *Handbook of Prescriptions for Emergency*, it also records the first aid methods of trauma (open wounds called "sores"), describes various methods of hemostasis of wounds, and the emergency treatment methods such as internal diseases, external diseases, injuries caused by various poisons, insects and animal. It's very rich in content. Meanwhile, the book also summarizes China's achievements in medical development since Jin Dynasty, such as detailed records of malaria types and symptoms and more than 30 prescriptions. The invention of artemisinin by the Chinese pharmacologist Tu Youyou, for which she won the Nobel Prize in Physiology or Medicine in 2015, was inspired by the description of the preparation method of "*Artemisia annua*" for treating malaria. It's recorded in the *Handbook of Prescriptions for Emergency* like this: "Take one grip of sweet wormwood herb, soak it in 2L (500g today) of water, then squeeze it into juice and drink it all." It can be seen that this book contains valuable treatment experience and medical data, which is worthy of our in-depth collation and exploration.

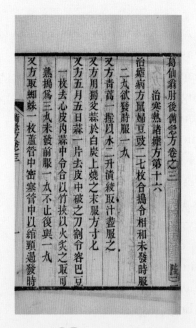

*Records of Artemisia annua in Handbook of*
*Prescriptions for Emergency*
(Zhǒu Hòu Bèi Jí Fāng，肘后备急方 )
now preserved in the Library of CACMS

## VI Huangfu Mi and the World's Earliest Acupuncture Monograph *A-B Classic of Acupuncture and Moxibustion*

Huangfu Mi (215–282 AD), whose young name is Jing, also called Shi'an and Xuan Yan. A native of Chaona County, Anding Prefecture (now Lingtai, Gansu Province), moved back to Xin'an (now Xin'an County, Henan Province). He was a scholar, medical scientist, and historian in the Western Jin Dynasty of the Three Kingdoms Period. He was born into a famous family in the Eastern Han Dynasty and was the great-grandson of Huangfu Song, a famous general in the Eastern Han Dynasty. Huangfu Mi played an influential role in the history of acupuncture and moxibustion, and was praised as "the originator of acupuncture and moxibustion" by later generations. After suffering from wind arthralgia at the age of 42, he began to study medicine and acupuncture, and then achieved great success. Referring to *Miraculous Pivot, Plain Questions*, and *Mingtang Hole Acupuncture Treatment Essentials*, Huangfu Mi "deleted its false, superfluous and repetitive words, and discussed its essence". In addition, he integrated his practice, tried countless times of needling himself, constantly revised and improved the acupuncture and moxibustion methods of human acupoints and meridians, and compiled *Three Acupuncture and Moxibustion Classics A and B of the Yellow Emperor*, also known as *A-B Classic of Acupuncture and Moxibustion, A-B Classic* and *Three Acupuncture and Moxibustion of the Yellow Emperor*.

*A-B Classic of Acupuncture and Moxibustion* is the earliest and most comprehensive acupuncture monograph in China. It consists of 12 volumes and 128 chapters. The first 6 volumes discuss the basic theories of acupuncture and acupoints, while the last 6 volumes record the treatment methods of various diseases, including etiology, pathogenesis, symptoms, diagnosis, acupoint selection, acupuncture, moxibustion, prognosis, etc. This book adopts the method of classification by meridians. Based on the summarization and absorption of the essence of some medical classics including *Miraculous Pivot, Plain Questions*, and *Mingtang Hole Acupuncture Treatment Essentials*, 349 acupoints were determined, which was 189 more than those mentioned in *Huangdi Neijing*. The meridial distribution and location of acupoints were defined, the names of acupoints were unified, and the correct names and aliases were distinguished. Meanwhile, 35 meridian routes were divided by the body parts and line (head, face, neck, chest, abdomen, limbs, etc.), and the indications and contraindications of each acupoint, needling depth, and numbers of moxi cones were described in detail.

The *A-B Classic of Acupuncture and Moxibustion* summarized the theories and clinical treatment experience of acupuncture and moxibustion before Jin Dynasty, which established norms for the development of acupuncture and moxibustion in the later generations and played a great role in the development of acupuncture and moxibustion. The acupuncture works from Jin to Song Dynasty, such as *Illustrated Classic of Acupoints on the Bronze Figure*, whose acupoints and indications are basically not beyond the scope of this book. *Classic of Nourishing Life with Acupuncture and Moxibustion* and other monographs were edited according to this book. *A Collection of Gems in Acupuncture and Moxibustion* and *The Great Compendium of Acupuncture and Moxibustion* in Ming and Qing Dynasties are based on this book. Since its publication, this book has received attention from the medical community and is regarded as a must-read book for medical students. As is said in *Essential Recipes for Emergent Use Worth A Thousand Gold–Great Medical Practice* recorded, "Anyone who wants to be a great doctor must know very well *Plain Questions, A-B Classic of Acupuncture and Moxibustion, Yellow Emperor Needle Classics*[①], *Mingtang Hole Acupuncture Treatment Essentials*, and other classics."

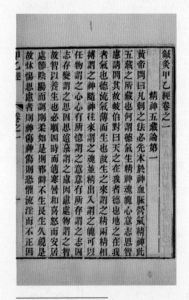

*Photoprint of Classic of A-B Classic of Acupuncture and Moxibustion*
(Zhēn Jiǔ Jiǎ Yǐ Jīng, 针灸甲乙经)
now preserved in the Library of CACMS

---

① i.e. *Miraculous Pivot*.

## VII Wang Shuhe and *Pulse Classic*

Wang Shuhe, named Xi, lived in Gaoping in the 3rd century. He was a famous medical scientist in Wei and Jin Dynasties and once served as an imperial physician. Gan Bozong of Tang Dynasty said in his *Record of Celebrated Doctors* that Wang Shuhe was "calm and knowledgeable, studying prescriptions and pulse, mastering in diagnosis and pulse-taking, grasping the ways of health maintenance, and deeply understanding theories of disease treatment". Wang Shuhe collected, sorted out, edited the collated writings of Zhang zhongjing, which were later corrected and published by Lin Yi and others in Song Dynasty, which is now *Treatise on Cold Pathogenic Disease*. Wang Shuhe himself professed, "I collected and sorted out Zhang zhongjing's theory, recorded its syndromes, pulse diagnosis, sensuality, and effective prescriptions to prevent unexpected diseases." This showed that the theories collated by Wang Shuhe were carried out from the aspects of pulse, syndrome, treatment, and prescription, which embodied Zhang Zhongjing's spirit of syndrome differentiation and treatment.

Wang Shuhe had a wealth of theoretical and clinical experience, especially in pulseology. In his clinical practice, he deeply realized the importance and complexity of pulse diagnosis. As pointed out in the preface to *Pulse Classic*, "Pulse is subtle, and it is difficult to distinguish." At the same time, it was considered that "in terms of pulse-taking, it is easy to learn, but difficult to identify different kinds of pulse in clinic". Sometimes pulse-taking was even metaphysicized or was not studied. The theory of pulse in *Huangdi Neijing* and the *Classic of Questioning*, which were handed down from ancient times, was profound and difficult to understand. At that time, there were no monographs on pulse. Therefore, Wang Shuhe devoted himself and finally wrote *Pulse Classic* based on summarizing the gist of ancient doctors' classics and recording pulse theory, combining his long-term clinical practice experience.

*Pulse Classic* consists of 10 volumes, 97 chapters, and about 100,000 words. It is the earliest monograph on pulseology in China, which is a collection of the remarkable achievements of pulseology before Wei and Jin Dynasties. In the book, the diagnostic method of "three positions and nine indicators" was updated to the method of "taking Cunkou alone". It systematically expounded on the aspects of standardizing pulse names, determining various pulse characteristics, and viscera belonging to cun-guan-chi, which made the pulse method systematic and standardized and dramatically promoted the development of TCM pulseology.

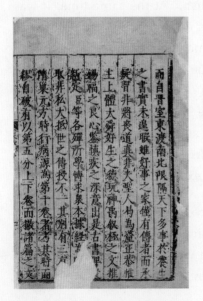

*Photoprint of Pulse Classic*
(Mài Jīng，脉经)
now preserved in the Library of CACMS

# VIII The Prime Minister Living in Seclusion and Famous Doctor—Tao Hongjing

Tao Hongjing (456–536 AD), courtesy-named Tongming, was a native of Moling, Danyang (now Nanjing, Jiangsu Province) in the Southern Liang Dynasty and called himself Huayang Hermit. He is a famous pharmacist, alchemist, and writer, known as the "Prime Minister living in seclusion". His works include the *Variorum of Shennong's Classic of Materia Medica, Medical Formulary of Golden Elixir Pill, General Formula of Medicine*, and so on.

Xiao Yan, Emperor Wu of Liang had been good friends with Tao Hongjing before he became emperor. When Xiao Yan initially won the power to prepare for the country's founding, he couldn't decide what name to use. According to the nursery rhymes circulating at that time and the books on predicting good or bad luck, Tao Hongjing said that the country name should be "水刃木处", which is a combination of the word "梁". Xiao Yan took his suggestion and entitled the country Liang. Afterward, Xiao Yan thanked Tao hongjing and sent people into the mountain to console him. According to the history books, Emperor Wu "continued to show kindness and courtesy to Tao Hongjing and kept sending him messages". Emperor Wu knew that Tao Hongjing was a prodigy and asked him to be an official on several occasions, but Tao turned down his offer. The emperor's imperial edict was urgent, so he drew two oxen and had them taken to the emperor. In the painting, one ox is among aquatic plants, while the other is added with a golden cage. Someone persistently drives it away with a whip. Seeing this, the emperor said with a smile, "This man has no desire for high position and great wealth. It seems that he intends to imitate the turtle crawling freely in the mud dragging its tail (From *Zhuangzi*, a metaphor for a life of freedom and seclusion). How can attract him?" He just sent someone to consult on military affairs. This is how the reputation of "the Prime Minister in seclusion" was formed.

Tao Hongjing made outstanding contributions to pharmacology, and he was the first person to systematize and creatively develop herbology. Tao Hongjing selected 365 new species from his *Miscellaneous Records of Famous Physicians* and added them to *Shennong's Classic of Materia Medica*, which increased the number of medicines from 365 to 730, and revised, adjusted, and annotated them one by one to compile the book *Variorum of Shennong's Classic of Materia Medica*. He was meticulous and rigorous when sorting out, respected the original work very much, didn't scribble or change the original work, nor did he make careless remarks. Even if there were supplements, he distinguished his statement from the original book's. When the 365 kinds of medicines he selected were co-edited with *Shennong's Classic of Materia Medica*, the contents of *Shennong's Classic of Materia Medica* and *Miscellaneous Records of Famous Physicians* were written in red and black, respectively. The practice he pioneered was followed by subsequent annotators. He pioneered the classification method of seven categories, including jade, vegetation, insects, animals, fruits, vegetables, rice, and famous but unused, which is still in use today. After systematic induction and summary, Tao Hongjing put forward the concept of "universal medicine for all diseases" for the first time. This inductive method combines the functions and indications of medicines with the characteristics of diseases, which is very suitable for clinical use.

The publication of the *Variorum of Shennong's Classic of Materia Medica* greatly influenced the development of TCM. *Newly Revised Materia Medica*—the first pharmacopoeia in the Tang Dynasty was further revised based on this book.

## IX Lei Xiao and *Master Lei's Discourse on Drug Processing*

With the discovery and application of TCM, the processing of Chinese materia medica came into being. Its history can be traced back to the primitive society. In history, processing is also called "paozhi", "zhizao", "xiuzhi" or "xiushi". There are some scattered records about the processing of medicinal materials in *Huangdi Neijing, Treatise on Febrile Diseases, Shennong's Classic of Materia Medica*, and *Handbook of Prescriptions for Emergency*. Before Sui and Tang Dynasties, doctors used medicines collected and processed on their own. Later, there were special pharmacies, and the processing of Chinese materia medica became a particular industry, which required the formulation of a set of technical standards and operational specifications to ensure efficacy. During the Southern and Northern Dynasties, Lei Xiao sorted out various processing methods of predecessors and compiled *Master Lei's Discourse on Drug Processing*, the first complete monograph on drug processing in China, for which Lei Xiao was also honored as the founder of Chinese medicinal processing.

Lei Xiao, whose life history is unknown, was first found in *History of the Sui Dynasty–Bibliography*. He, also known as Lei Gong, did a lot of research on drug processing. There are three volumes of *Master Lei's Discourse on Drug Processing* (also known as *Pao Zhi Fang*), which contains 300 kinds of medicines. It introduces processing, identification, and cutting, mastery of high and low flames, selection of auxiliary materials, and processing methods. In addition, the basic knowledge of storage, processing, and taboos of Chinese herbal pieces was also introduced. In the original book, "seventeen methods of processing" were systematically summarized, including baking, broiling, simmering, stir-frying, calcining, refining, exposure to the sun, grinding in water, and other common methods, which are highly practical. Some pharmaceutical methods and medicine selection requirements in the book still have practical influence and are regarded as classic guidelines for processing TCM by later generations.

*Master Lei's Discourse on Drug Processing* is the first summary of the processing technology of TCM in Chinese history, and it is also an important document for the identification of TCM. Its original work was lost but was still handed down thanks to the writings of later doctors works. This book had a great influence on the development of pharmacology in later generations. Famous monographs on Chinese medicine processing, such as Li Zhongzi's *Lei Gong's Medicine Processing* and Miao Xiyong's *Traditional Chinese Medicine Processing in Ming Dynasty* were all based on sorting out *Master Lei's Discourse on Drug Processing* and the collection of some folk experience. Nowadays, the processing of TCM still refers to the theory in the original book, which plays a vital role in improving efficacy, slowing down toxicity, harmonizing dosage forms, and facilitating medication.

# Chapter 3

## Sui and Tang Dynasties

—Diversified Development of TCM

Sui and Tang Dynasties were the most prosperous period of Chinese feudal society, and Tang Dynasty was the most glorious chapter in the long history of the Chinese nation. During this period, a strong national strength, enlightened politics, prosperous economy, advanced science and technology, cultural diversity, and ethnic harmony provided a good foundation for the development and dissemination of TCM. Based on the all-around development of medical theory, pharmacology, Chinese medical formulas and clinical disciplines, there is a trend of summarizing and compiling TCM. The unprecedentedly comprehensive medical classics and prescriptions in history appeared in this period. Besides, the compilation level of literature collation, pharmacological works, and summary monographs of clinical disciplines made significant progress, which had an important impact on the later medicine.

# I The Earliest National Medical School—Imperial Medical Academy

In the thousands of years of Chinese history, Sui Dynasty lasted for only less than 40 years, but it greatly influenced Chinese history and civilization development. The Sui Dynasty unified the division which lasted for nearly 300 years, initiated the imperial examination, and opened the Beijing-Hangzhou Grand Canal and established the world's earliest "National Medical School"— the government-run Imperial Medical Academy, which greatly influenced the development of TCM in later generations.

Emperor Yang in the Sui Dynasty attached great importance to medicine. With his promotion, TCM in the Sui Dynasty made new progress. During his reign, Department of Chancellors was changed into Ministry of Internal Affairs to take charge of the Administration of Medicine. He personally organized and compiled *Four Seas Gathering Prescriptions* (2,600 volumes) and a simplified version of *Four Seas Gathering List* (300 volumes), which systematically summarized the medical prescriptions of the past. The Imperial Medical Academy founded by him was not only the highest official medical education institution in the world at that time, but also assumed certain medical management functions. According to *History of the Sui Dynasty–Officials Records*, "Minister of Ceremonies is in charge of two entitled Minister of Imperial Medical Academy and one director, and the Imperial Medical Academy has two people in charge of medicine, 200 doctors, two medicinal gardeners, two teaching assistants, two massage doctors and two incantation masters."

The Tang Dynasty followed the Sui system and established the Imperial Medical Academy. Compared with Sui Dynasty, the Imperial Medical Academy of Tang Dynasty had a new development. First, it has a larger scale with nearly 400 staff members; second, department division is more detailed, mainly including pharmacology, medicine and administration, and each department is subdivided according to its functions; third, there is a clear academic system, such as a seven-year academic system for internal medicine, a five-year academic system for surgery and pediatrics, and a four-year academic system for ENT; fourth, there were full-time management positions available. In the curriculum of the Imperial Medical Academy, students were required to "be adept at" the classic basic courses of TCM, such as *The Yellow Emperor's Mingtang Moxibustion Classic*, *Plain Questions*, *Yellow Emperor Needle Classics* , and *Shennong's Classic of Materia Medica*. After the completion of basic courses, students begin to receive specialized education. Medical students who are excellent in academic performance could be assigned to work in advance, and those who fail will be demoted for no more than two years. Otherwise, they will be removed. The curriculum of the Imperial Medical Academy not only pays attention to the study of classical theory but also practical operation. The curriculum also includes the planting, cultivation, collection, and storage of Chinese medicinals, which requires medical students to know all kinds of herbs and their medicinal properties. This education mode broke the single teacher-apprentice mode of TCM education at that time, and trained many outstanding talents. Chao Yuanfang, a famous doctor, was a medical doctor of the Imperial Medical Academy.

The Imperial Medical Academy in the Tang Dynasty is the earliest medical school in the world, more than 200 years earlier than the earliest medical school in Europe, Salerno School of Medicine, Italy (846 AD). The government of Tang Dynasty offered medical education in the central government, and in every state, which was the significant progress in the development of medical education in ancient China and had a positive impact on medical education in later generations.

## II The First Monograph on Etiology and Syndromes—*General Treatise on Causes and Manifestations of All Diseases*

In 610 AD, the Sui government organized Chao Yuanfang, a doctor of the imperial medicine academy, and others to edit *General Treatise on Causes and Manifestations of All Diseases*. This book is the first monograph systematically discussing etiology and syndromes in Chinese history. It comprehensively sorts out and summarizes the understanding of clinical syndromes since Qin and Han Dynasties, deeply analyzes and studies the etiology of various diseases, and puts forward many original ideas, which has greatly influenced the development of medicine in later generations.

There are 50 volumes and 67 sections in the *General Treatise on Causes and Manifestations of All Diseases* which contains 1,739 treatises on the etiology and syndromes. Its main contributions and achievements in Chinese medicine include the following aspects:

First, it enriched the content of TCM theory by breaking through the predecessors' general theory of "three types of disease causes" in etiology theory. For example, the pathogens of scabies and other diseases were confirmed in the book. Through clinical observation, Chao Yuanfang pointed out that "There are several kinds of scabies and all have worms" , "Scabies often occur on hands and feet, and even throughout the body", "There are all insects, and people often pick them with a needle, like a worm inside water. This is caused by the pathogenic wind heat on the skin". It can be seen that the book has a comprehensive and correct understanding of the scabies pathogen, its infectivity, location, and the essentials of diagnosis, which is more than 1,000 years earlier than a report on the study of sarcoptic mite in Europe in 1758 AD.

Second, Chao accurately described the syndromes and clinical manifestations of various diseases through long-term practical observation. Such as in the discussion of chest obstruction, it was believed that "The cold pathogenic qi is in the zang-fu viscera. When the body is in a deficiency state, the cold pathogenic qi rushes upward to the chest and becomes chest discomfort", and its initial clinical manifestations are "stuffiness, choking, dry and ithchy throat, salivary dryness", and worst manifestations are "The chest is hard, full and with acute pain, the muscles are painful and cramped like pins and needles. The patient cannot lie on the stomach, and the skin in front of his/ her chest hurts so that it can't be touched with hands. His/her chest is full with shortness of breath. Coughing and spitting causes pain. There is fidget, spontaneous sweating, or heartache radiating to the back". The book also records the clinical manifestations of leprosy, stroke, jaundice, gonorrhea, diabetes, and other diseases in detail, which shows that Chinese medicine doctors had a systematic understanding of these diseases more than 1,300 years ago.

In addition, many surgical methods and suture techniques for treating trauma were recorded in *General Treatise on Causes and Manifestations of All Diseases*. For example, in the chapter Golden Sore and Intestinal Breakage, it is stated, "if one has an intestinal breakage with metal-inflicted wounds, the degree of disease should be given attention to. It can be reconnected quickly if the intestines are seen at both ends. First use a needled to suture. Then chicken blood is smeared over the suture area to prevent intestinal leakage, and finally push it inside." The discussion of theoretical principles, operation methods and postoperative precautions in suturing broken intestines is still of reference significance today. The techniques contained in the book, such as treating abdominal trauma, excising greater omentum, ligating blood vessels to stop bleeding, and removing foreign bodies from trauma, reflect the important achievements of clinical medicine in the 7th century in China.

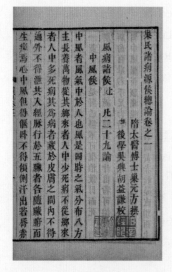

*Photoprint of General Treatise on Causes and Manifestations of All Diseases*
(Zhū Bìng Yuán Hòu Lùn, 诸病源候论 )
now preserved in the Library of CACMS

# III The King of Medicine Sun Simiao and *Recipes Worth A Thousand Gold Pieces*

Sun Simiao (581–682 AD) was a native of Huayuan, Jingzhao, in the Tang Dynasty (now Yaozhou District, Tongchuan City, Shaanxi Province). He was a great medical scientist who was talented and rigorous in his studies. He was also a great scholar who rolled Taoism, Buddhism, and Confucianism into one. Sun Simiao had been engaged in clinical practice for 80 years and had made indelible contributions to the development of TCM. He is honored as the "King of Medicine" by later generations.

According to the *Old Book of Tang*, Dugu Xin, the minister of the Western Wei Dynasty, regarded highly of Sun Simiao and called him a "wonder child". When he was 18, Sun Simiao was determined to become a doctor. "He had a sense of understanding about medicine, so he was able to help many of my neighbors and friends who were suffering from illnesses and diseases." At the age of 20, he began to treat his neighbors with good effect. After, he studied ancient medical books more diligently such as *Huangdi Neijing, Treatise on Cold Pathogenic and Miscellaneous Diseases, Shennong's Classic of Materia Medica* and collected folk formulas, sought folk treatment experience, enthusiastically treated people, and accumulated many valuable clinical experiences. Given the complicated and scattered ancient medical formulas and complex retrieval, Sun Simiao collected the theories of various medical schools, then deleted the identical and simplified them. Furthermore, combined his own clinical experience, he wrote medical works *Essential Recipes for Emergent Use Worth A Thousand Gold Pieces* and *A Supplement to Recipes Worth a Thousand Gold Pieces*, referred to as *Recipes Worth A Thousand Gold Pieces (Qianjin Fang)* for short. Among them, *Essential Recipes for Emergent Use Worth A Thousand Gold Pieces* was written before Sun Simiao was 70 years old, and *A Supplement to Recipes Worth A Thousand Gold Pieces* was written in his later years, which supplemented the former. *Recipes Worth A Thousand Gold Pieces* records in detail the medical theories, formulas, diagnostic methods, treatment methods, health preservation, daoyin, and other aspects of major medical works before the Tang Dynasty, among which more than 6,500 medical formulas are collected, and more than 800 kinds of medicines are recorded, which can be called the first encyclopedia of clinical medicine in Chinese history. The achievement of *Recipes Worth A Thousand Gold Pieces* represents the highest level of medical development in the prosperous Tang Dynasty. It has significant influence in China, is widely spread in Asian countries, and is praised as "the treasure of mankind" by Japanese medical community.

Sun Simiao is not only a clinical master but also attaches great importance to the cultivation of medical ethics. Emperor Taizong and Gaozong of Tang Dynasty both called Sun Simiao into Chang'an, and conferred him a title, but he turned their offer down. However, he never refused when ordinary people asked him to treat diseases. He stressed: "Whenever a great doctor treats diseases, he must calm his nerves, have no desire, and first show great compassion and vow to save the patients. If some people come for help because of illness, we should not consider their status, wealth, age, beauty or ugliness, close relation or not, Han nationality or ethnic minority, foolish or wise people. They all should be treated as our relatives." His noble medical ethics has been praised by later generations, and his view of "Virtual of Great Doctor" is still a classic that we study when we carry out medical ethics education.

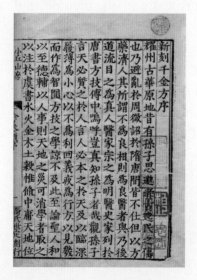

*Photoprint of Recipes Worth A Thousand Gold Pieces*
(Qiān Jīn Fāng, 千金方 )
now preserved in the Library of CACMS

## IV The First Pharmacopeia Issued by the Government—*Newly Revised Materia Medica*

With the rapid development of the social economy and transportation in the Tang Dynasty, materia medica knowledge gradually accumulated and enriched, and many new medicines and foreign medicines appeared, which expanded the field of materia medica knowledge. In 657 AD, Li Zhi, Emperor Gaozong of the Tang Dynasty, adopted Su Jing's suggestion to revise materia medica and recruited more than 20 famous medical scientists and administrative officials to do the work together and *Newly Revised Materia Medica* was compiled in 659 AD. This is the first pharmacopeia issued by the government in China and the earliest pharmacopeia in the world, more than 800 years earlier than the *Nuremberg Pharmacopoeia* in Europe (issued in 1542 AD).

The original book of *Newly Revised Materia Medica* consists of 54 volumes, including three parts: illustration, explanation of illustration, and materia medica. It contains 844 medicines, which are divided into 9 categories according to their natural attributes, such as jade, grass, wood, animals, insects and fish, fruits, vegetables, rice and grain, and famous but not used. In the compilation of this book, the Tang government extensively solicited opinions from all sides, emphasizing "consulting the public" and "determining the gains and losses in the group". During the period, all parts of the country were also ordered to send genuine regional medcinals produced locally as physical specimens for description. The materia medica part of the book supplements the medicines not recorded in ancient books, revises the incorrect contents, and introduces the nature, taste, origin, efficacy, indications, and collection time in detail. The illustration is drawn based on the extensive collection of medicinal materials from all over the country. In addition to the description of the configuration of medicinal materials, there are also medicine collection and processing contents.

*Newly Revised Materia Medica* systematically summarized the materia medica achievements before the Tang Dynasty, with rich illustrations and contents, and had high academic level and scientific value. Soon after the publication of this book, it was circulated all over the country. At that time, the Imperial Medical Academy, the highest medical authority in China, immediately used it as teaching material. *Newly Revised Materia Medica* also had a great influence abroad, and it was introduced to Japan shortly after its promulgation. In 701 AD, the medical law *Taiho Code–Physician Law* formulated by Japan listed *Newly Revised Materia Medica* as a compulsory book for medical students with 310 days of the study hours. The original work is now incomplete, and the volumes of illustration and explanation of illustration have all been lost. There are only photocopies and shadow copies of the fragmentary volumes of materia medica, and the content of *Newly Revised Materia Medica* is basically preserved because of the reference of later materia medica books and prescription books.

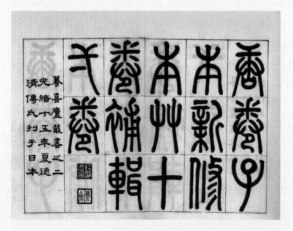

*Photoprint of Newly Revised Materia Medica*
(Xīn Xiū Běn Cǎo, 新修本草 )
now preserved in the Library of CACMS

# V A Masterpiece of Tibetan Medicine—*Four Medical Tantras*

Tibetan medicine is an integral part of TCM, and its theoretical system was formed in the Tubo Dynasty (that is, the 7th–9th century AD). At that time, the Tibet Dynasty and Tang Dynasty had frequent exchanges in the fields of politics, economy, culture, medicine, and health, which positively influenced the formation and development of Tibetan medicine. In this context, *Four Tantras* (Tibetan name *Jvxi*) was written by Tibetan medical scientist Yudho Yundan Gompo (708–833 AD). This book is the foundation work of Tibetan medicine, which laid the foundation for the formation of the Tibetan medical system. Yudho Yundan Gompo was honored as a "medical sage" by generations of Tibetan doctors because of his important contributions to the development of Tibetan medicine.

The *Four Tantras* is written in a similar style to the *Huangdi Neijing*, which is written in a seven-character or nine-character verse in the form of answering questions by the king of medicine. The whole book has 240,000 words and 156 chapters. This book is composed of four parts: the first part is *Zhajv*, or *General Principles*, which is the general medical theory; the second part is *Xiejv*, or *Discussion*, which tells about human anatomy, physiology, etiology, pathology, medicines, instruments, treatment principles, etc; the third part is *Men'ajv*, or *Secrets*, which is a theory of clinical diseases, and records of the clinical manifestations, diagnosis and treatment of various diseases; the fourth part is *Qinmajv*, or *Follow-up Collection*, which supplements pulse diagnosis and urine diagnosis, and introduces the processing and usage of medicines. After completing the *Four Tantras*, Tibetan medicine experts also added 79 color pictures composed of thousands of small pictures to illustrate the text contents including human anatomy and embryo, animals, plants, and minerals, various medical instruments, urine diagnosis, pulse diagnosis, food hygiene, disease prevention, etc. The existing color illustrations of the *Four Tantras*, drawn in the late Ming and early Qing Dynasties, are precious medical cultural relics.

*Four Tantras* comprehensively and systematically summarized the theory and practical experience of ancient Tibetan medicine, reflecting many unique features of Tibetan medicine. It is one of the most well-preserved and influential representatives of traditional medical classics at present. It represents the highest medical level in Tibet at that time, embodies the early humanities, history, tradition, literature, art, and crafts in Tibet, and has been translated into English, German, Mongolian, Japanese, Russian, and other languages. *Four Medical Tantras* had great influence on the world culture at that time, which is also considered an important literature with great research value to this day.

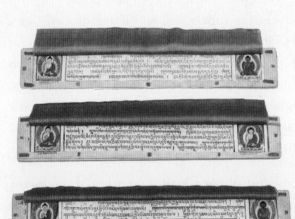

*Illustration on the inner page of Zhatang edition of Four Medical Tantras*
(Sì Bù Yī Diǎn, 四部医典)
engraved in 1546 AD

## VI Lin Daoren and the Great Work of TCM Orthopedics and Traumatology *Secrets of Treating Wounds and Bonesetting*

Orthopedics and traumatology had a long history in China, as early as the Zhou Dynasty, "sore and wound doctors" were responsible for dealing with "sores and wounds" and "fractures". In the barracks of the Han Dynasty, there were medical records "Orthopedics Book", which specially recorded the fractures of officers and soldiers, and there were also discussions on the medical technology of orthopedics and traumatology in various medical books. *Secrets of Treating Wounds and Bonesetting* written at the end of the Tang Dynasty, is the first existing monograph on orthopedics and traumatology in China and plays a critical role in the development history of orthopedics and traumatology in China.

Lin Daoren (about 790–850 AD), a native of Chang'an (now Xi'an, Shaanxi Province), surnamed Lin and given-name unknown, was a medical monk in the Tang Dynasty. According to historical records, Emperor Wuzong of Tang Dynasty issued an imperial edict to abolish Buddhism, ordering more than 260,000 Buddhist monks and nuns to resume secular life. Also, he engaged in agricultural and mulberry production, recovered thousands of hectares of temple fields, and returned them to the people. It was against this background that Lin Daoren left Chang'an and came to Zhong Village, Yichun County, Jiangxi Province, and unreservedly imparted his medical skills and the osteopathic book *Treating Wounds and Bonesetting* to an older man surnamed Peng, who often helped him cultivate. After his medical skills were passed on, Lin Daoren went to another place to live in seclusion. When people found that he suddenly disappeared, they said he was a celestial being and renamed the book *Secrets of Treating Wounds and Bonesetting*.

Lin's academic thought originated from the theory of qi and blood in *Huangdi Neijing* and *Classic of Questioning*. He inherited the experience and achievements of orthopedics and traumatology in *Handbook of Prescriptions for Emergency*, *Essential Recipes for Emergent Use Worth A Thousand Gold Pieces* and *Arcane Essentials from the Imperial Library*, forming a general treatment method featuring restoration, fixation, activity, internal and external medication, which initially laid the foundation for syndrome differentiation, method establishment, prescription and medication in orthopedics and traumatology. It enabled the principle of treatment based on syndrome differentiation of TCM to be applied to orthopedics and traumatology.

*Secrets of Treating Wounds and Bonesetting* is composed of three parts: "processing for treating bone injuries", "recipes" and "discourse on the recipes of treating injuries". For the first time, the book systematically formulated the treatment routine of fracture, dislocation and other injuries, including 14 steps such as local irrigation, diagnosis, traction, reduction, dressing and splint fixation. For fracture reduction and fixation, the treatment principle of "combination of activity with inertia" was put forward, and the surgical operation, manual reduction principles and treatment techniques of complex fractures are discussed in detail. In the process of manual reduction or surgical reduction, the application of anesthetics is emphasized. These treatment principles and methods still have a high theoretical level and clinical application value.

# VII Wang Tao and *Arcane Essentials from the Imperial Library*

Wang Tao (about 670–755 AD), a native of Mei county (now Mei County, Shaanxi Province), is a famous doctor in the Tang Dynasty and the great-grandson of Wang Mei, the prime minister of the Tang Dynasty. He had been sickly since childhood and often took medication treatment, so he developed a strong interest in medicine. Wang Tao once served as the governor of Sima in Xuzhou and Ye County. Later, he worked in Hongwen Library of the Royal Library of the Tang Dynasty for more than 20 years. As a result, he was able to read extensively and collect various medical prescriptions. The *Arcane Essentials from the Imperial Library*, *General Treatise on Causes and Manifestations of All Diseases*, and *Recipes Worth A Thousand Gold Pieces* were hailed as "three medical masterpieces" in Sui and Tang Dynasties by later generations. His *Arcane Essentials from the Imperial Library* drew on the strengths of many schools and made outstanding contributions to preserving the original appearance of ancient medical books and summarizing the medical achievements before the Tang Dynasty, which has been widely circulated in later generations.

*Arcane Essentials from the Imperial Library* was completed in 752 AD. It consists of 40 volumes, 1,104 subjects, and 6,000 prescriptions. The contents include: wind, surgery, bone, gynecology, obstetrics, pediatrics, psychosis, dermatology, ophthalmology, dentistry, and other subjects. Each chapter is described in an orderly manner. Among them, the theory part is mainly based on Chao Yuanfang's *General Treatise on Causes and Manifestations of All Diseases*, and the content of *Recipes Worth A Thousand Gold Pieces* is the most selected part of medical prescriptions. A large number of medical documents before Tang Dynasty were collated and preserved in the book, and the cited materials were marked with titles and volumes for easy checking. This writing style also set a good example for the collation of medical documents for later generations. A large number of folk recipes and experiential prescriptions were collected in the book, all of which detailed their therapeutic effect, treatment scope and source. In addition, there were new developments in the understanding of diseases in *Arcane Essentials from the Imperial Library*. For example, the book describes diabetes as "at every onset, the patient has a sweet urine", more than 900 years earlier than diabetes was recognized in Wales in 1670. The gold needle extraction (a traditional technique) for cataracts recorded in the book is the earliest in Chinese history, and is still used in clinical practice today.

After the *Arcane Essentials from the Imperial Library* was published, it was quickly circulated in Korea, Japan and other countries, and the *New Book of Tang* praised it as the "World Treasure". "If one person never reads the prescriptions of *Arcane Essentials from the Imperial Library* and the theory of *Recipes Worth A Thousand Gold Pieces*, he/she doesn't read extensively, nor is his/her medication magical." This shows the high status of this book in the medical field and Wang Tao is also known as the master of literature collation.

# Chapter 4

## Song, Jin and Yuan Dynasties

—Academic Contending and Achievements of TCM

The Song, Jin, and Yuan Dynasties witnessed the rapid development of TCM with various schools and achievements, which greatly influenced the development of TCM in later generations. Especially in the Northern Song Dynasty, many emperors, such as the Song Emperors Taizu, Taizong, Renzong, and Huizong, attached great importance to TCM and issued several edicts to develop medicine. With the organization and promotion of the government, medical exchange among ethnic groups were frequent and medical and political facilities were constantly improved. Besides, Chinese materia medica, Chinese medical formulas, acupuncture and moxibustion, and clinical sciences were developing rapidly. Many classic works on TCM were compiled by the official organization, and standardized research on prescriptions, patent medicines and meridians, and acupoints became a common practice, leaving a deep impression on the history of TCM.

# I The Establishment of Medical Literature Correction Bureau in Song Dynasty

TCM was consistently implemented as a "benevolent governance" by ancient emperors, and the emperors of the Song Dynasty attached great importance to and supported the development of TCM, among which 830 medical edicts were issued in the Northern Song Dynasty. For example, in the fourth year of Kaibao (971 AD), Zhao Kuangyin, Emperor Taizu of Song Dynasty, issued the Imperial Edict on Visiting Elders with Excellent Medical Skills to select medical talents from all over the country to enrich the Imperial Medical Academy. In the sixth year of Taipingxingguo (981 AD), Zhao Jiong, Emperor Taizong of Song Dynasty issued the Imperial Edict on Visiting and Seeking Medical Books, collecting medical books all over the country, and awarding them official positions or materials according to how many books they presented. In the fourth year of Tiansheng (1026 AD), Zhao Zhen, Emperor Renzong of Song Dynasty, once more collected and revised medical books, and ordered medical scientists and bibliographers to sort them out. At the same time, the progress and development of printing and papermaking also created good conditions for the printing and dissemination of medical books. Under this background, "Medical Literature Correction Bureau" was set up by the Song Dynasty government in 1057 AD, gathering a group of famous scholars and doctors at that time, such as Zhang Yuxi, Lin Yi, Gao Baoheng, Sun Zhao, Qin Zonggu et al, to collect, collate and sort out medical books of the past dynasties.

The establishment of the Medical Literature Correction Bureau is pioneering work in the history of the development of TCM. Han Qi and Fan Zhongyan, who were recommended by the Medical Literature Correction Bureau successively, were all influential scholars at that time. In the preface of the corrected medical books, Lin Yi et al repeatedly mentioned the specific requirements of Emperors Renzong and Yingzong of Song to the Medical Literature Correction Bureau. Namely, "Renzong thought that the ancestor's legacy would be forgotten if there were no policies. Renzong issued an edict to inform the scholars to make corrections. We temporarily served as the officer of proofreading. After a year of self-examination, we searched the official and private collections, collected numerous books, and gradually searched for their meaning, and corrected their mistakes." "The state ordered scholar-born ministers to correct medical books, and ordered them to take *Plain Questions*, *Jiu Xu* (Another version of *Miraculous Pivot*), *Miraculous Pivot*, *Grand Simplicity*, *Essential Recipes for Emergent Use Worth A Thousand Gold Pieces*, *A Supplement to Recipes Worth a Thousand Gold Pieces* and *Arcane Essentials from the Imperial Library* for proofreading." It can be seen from the various descriptions in the books that the emperors of the Song Dynasty attached great importance to the examination and approval of medical classics and ancient medical books.

After the establishment of the Medical Literature Correction Bureau, it took more than 10 years to complete the correction and publication of 10 most representative medical masterpieces before the Song Dynasty, such as *Plain Questions*, *Treatise on Cold Pathogenic Disease*, *Synopsis of Golden Chamber*, *The Canon of the Golden Chamber and Jade Sheath*, *A-B Classic of Acupuncture and Moxibustion*, *Pulse Classic*, *General Treatise on Causes and Manifestations of All Diseases*, *Essential Recipes for Emergent Use Worth A Thousand Gold Pieces*, *A Supplement to Recipes Worth a Thousand Gold Pieces*, and *Arcane Essentials from the Imperial Library*. All of these made a significant contribution to the development of TCM in the Song Dynasty and the dissemination of medical books to future generations.

## II The Achievements and Values of *Taiping Holy Prescriptions for Universal Relief*

*Taiping Holy Prescriptions for Universal Relief* is a large prescription book issued by the government after *Recipes Worth A Thousand Gold Pieces* and *Arcane Essentials from the Imperial Library* in the Tang Dynasty. The book records in detail the prescription books before the Northern Song Dynasty and the folk recipes at that time, which greatly influenced the development of TCM formulas, and also has a lot of discussion and elaboration on medical theories.

*Taiping Holy Prescriptions for Universal Relief* was compiled by Wang Huaiyin, a medical scientist in Northern Song Dynasty, under the edict of Emperor Taizong of Song. Wang Huaiyin, a native of Suiyang, Songzhou (now Shangqiu, Henan Province), was a Taoist priest at the beginning, proficient in TCM and skilled in medical skills. Before Emperor Taizong of Song Dynasty ascended the throne, he often discussed medical principles with him. After Emperor Taizong ascended the throne, he was made to secularize and appointed as Physician Serving the Royalty, and later promoted to medical officers of Hanlin Medical Official Academy. In 978 AD, Emperor Taizong of Song Dynasty ordered the official doctors of the Imperial Academy to compile a prescription book, and organized famous doctors from all over the country to engage in this work in the form of government. After nationwide survey and collection, the compilation lasted for 14 years and this book was completed in 992 AD. After completing *Taiping Holy Prescriptions for Universal Relief*, Emperor Taizong of Song Dynasty gave the title of the book and made the preface himself, which shows his concern and attention to this book.

*Taiping Holy Prescriptions for Universal Relief* consists of 100 volumes, 1,670 subjects, and 16,834 formulas, including pulse method, formula medication, syndromes and diseases of five zang organs, internal and external injuries, orthopedics and traumatology, incised (metal-inflicted) wound, obstetrics, gynecology and children, as well as pellet, dietetic therapy, tonifying, acupuncture, moxibustion, and so on. The first part of each subject contains the discussions of etiology, pathology and syndromes in *General Treatise on Causes and Manifestations of All Diseases*, followed by the corresponding formulas and therapies. The book emphasizes that doctors must identify yin and yang, deficiency and excess, cold and heat, and exterior and interior in the treatment first. Then, they should ensure the formula is given with the syndrome and the medicine is applied with the formula. Moreover, it discusses the relationship between etiology, pathogenesis, syndrome and formulas and medicines, which embodies the complete treatment based on syndrome differentiation system of theory, method, formula and medicine. There are many kinds of medicines selected, and some of them are seldom used or even not used by predecessors.

*Taiping Holy Prescriptions for Universal Relief* is the first prescription book written by the state in the history of China, which is voluminous and rich in content. It is a complete collection of theory, method, formula, and medicine, which is of great value to collate and study TCM. As a masterpiece of collection of medical formulas before the Song Dynasty, it was highly respected by doctors of all ages and widely cited. It was also circulated in Korea and Japan, and the *Integration Prescription of Rural Medicine*, written in the early Li Dynasty of Korea quoted extensively from this book.

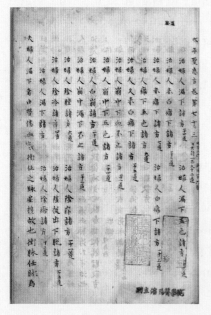

*Photoprint of Taiping Holy Prescriptions for Universal Relief*
(Tài Píng Shèng Huì Fāng，太平圣惠方)
now preserved in the Library of CACMS

# III Wang Weiyi and Bronze Acupuncture Figure

Wang Weiyi (about 987–1067 AD), also known as Weide, was a medical officer in the Northern Song Dynasty and a famous acupuncturist. He used to be a medical officer of Hanlin Medical Official Academy, a medical research institution and served as a Physician in the Department of Internal Affairs. He has profound research on acupuncture theory, technique, illustrated classics in ancient medical books. By the imperial edict of Emperor Renzong of the Song Dynasty, Wang Weiyi sorted out the contents of acupuncture and moxibustion in the books of the previous dynasties and completed the *Illustrated Classic of Acupoints on the Bronze Figure* in 1206 AD. After reading it, Emperor Renzong of the Song Dynasty thought, "Although the exegesis of the classics is fine, if the scholars stick to it but are not flexible, they will make mistakes." Also, he pointed out, "It is better to see with your own eyes than to understand with your heart; it is better to take actions directly than to explain with theory." Further, he also ordered, "Cast a bronze acupuncture figure as a model. There are five viscera and six organs in its body and water or mercury is injected into the meridians and acupoints of the whole body. If the silver needle can pierce into the relevant acupoints on the meridians, water will come out. The corresponding acupoints are marked with names so that the viewer clearly understands the location of the meridian and acupoints and those who have doubts immediately have their confusion resolved." According to the emperor's request, Wang Weiyi cast two bronze acupuncture figures in 1027 AD. At that time, this pair of bronze acupuncture figures were first used for teaching in imperial medical institutions, and second, they were used to assess the acupuncture skills of doctors.

According to literature records, one of the bronze acupuncture figures designed and cast by Wang Weiyi was placed in the Hanlin Medical Official Academy and the other in Renji Hall of Daxiangguo Temple. The height of the bronze figure is close to that of a normal adult, and the front and back sides of the bronze figure can be opened and closed. The internal organs are carved into the body, which is basically similar to the size and position of the human body. There are acupoints engraved on the surface of the bronze status, and the names of acupoints are engraved beside them. The cavities are sealed with yellow wax and injected with water (or mercury). If the acupoint selection is accurate, the needle enters and the water exits; if the acupoint selection is inaccurate, the needle will not enter.

It is said that during the war between Song and Jin Dynasties, people of the Jin used to ask for the bronze acupuncture figures as a negotiation condition, which shows their preciousness. After the Yuan Dynasty set its capital in Beijing, this pair of bronze figures were moved from Kaifeng, Henan Province to Beijing. In 1265 AD, the Nepalese craftsman Anika trimmed the bronze acupuncture figures. In the Ming Dynasty, Zhu Qizhen, Emperor Yingzong of the Ming Dynasty, organized metalworkers to cast copper to imitate the bronze figures because he saw the holes and the meridians of the bronze statues cast by Wang Weiyi were dim and indistinguishable. However, after years of war, the bronze acupuncture status of the Song Dynasty disappeared. Since the advent of bronze acupuncture figures in the Song Dynasty, bronze statues' casting had developed from official to folk. From the Ming Dynasty, there were more than 100 official or individual imitations of bronze acupuncture figures.

Since ancient times, acupuncture and moxibustion therapy has been widely used in the treatment of diseases and health preservation. Accurate acupoint positioning is vital for the application and curative effect of acupuncture and moxibustion. As a model of acupuncture teaching in ancient China, bronze acupuncture figures played an important role in the development of acupuncture and moxibustion.

## IV The First Monograph on Pediatrics of TCM—*Key to Therapeutics of Children's Diseases*

The research on pediatrics existed for a long time in ancient China, but there was no monograph on pediatric diseases in an all-round way. It was not until Song Dynasty that Qian Yi, a famous medical scientist, wrote *Key to Therapeutics of Children's Diseases*, which systematically summarized the treatment of children based on syndrome differentiation for the first time and made the development of pediatrics of TCM reach a new height. Since then, it has become an independent specialized discipline.

Qian Yi (1032–1113 AD), courtesy-named Zhongyang, whose ancestral home is Qiantang, Zhejiang Province, moved north to Yunzhou, Dongping (now Dongping County, Shandong Province) with his grandfather. Qian Yi lost his mother in childhood. His father Qian Hao was good at medicine. However, he liked drinking and traveling. When Qian Yi was three years old, his father traveled east to the sea and did not return. Later, Qian Yi studied medicine with his uncle Lv, specializing in pediatrics. He worked hard, learned knowledge of various schools, and he was famous then. During the Yuanfeng period of Emperor Shenzong of Song Dynasty, Qian Yi went to the Bianliang (now Kaifeng, Henan Province) to practice medicine and gained great fame in the capital. Because he cured the complex diseases of Princess Royal and Prince Yi Guogong, he was appointed by Emperor Shenzong of Song Dynasty as an imperial medical officer. Qian Yi accumulated rich experience in the clinic for decades. He combined this experience with classic medical works such as *Huangdi Neijing, Treatise on Cold Pathogenic and Miscellaneous Diseases, Shennong's Classic of Materia Medica,* and other theories. Then, he wrote a pediatric monograph—*Key to Therapeutics of Children's Diseases*, which was compiled, summarized, proofread, and edited by his disciple Yan Jizhong. It was officially published in the first year of Xuanhe of the Song Dynasty (1119 AD). The book consists of 3 volumes. The first volume discusses the treatment method and pulse syndrome and includes more than 80 common pediatric diseases; 23 cases are discussed in the second volume; the third volume is on various formulas, and 124 formulas are listed. The treatment of the whole book follows the physiological and pathological characteristics of "the zang-fu of a child is weak, and it is easy to be deficient and excessive, cold and heat", and the formula is moderate in cold and warmth, combined with tonifying and reducing, reinforcing healthy qi to eliminate pathogenic factors based on softening and nourishing zang-fu. The book details Qian Yi's method of "syndrome differentiation of five zang organs", which is suitable for children, and records Qian Yi's innovative methods of facial inspection "facial syndrome" and intraocular inspection "intraocular syndrome", namely, the diagnosis method of examining children's diseases of five zang organs from face and eyes. In addition, many formulas recorded in the book, such as Yigong Powder, Liuwei Dihuang Pill, Shengma Gegen Decoction, Daochi Powder, etc., are still widely used in pediatric clinics.

*Key to Therapeutics of Children's Diseases* is the first existing pediatric monograph in China. The *Bibliography of Imperial Collection of Four Divisions* commented, "Children's classical formulas are rare through the ages, and pediatrics has been specialized since Qian Yi, and his book is also the originator of pediatrics." Qian Yi is also honored as "the saint of pediatrics" because of his important contribution to the development of pediatrics of TCM.

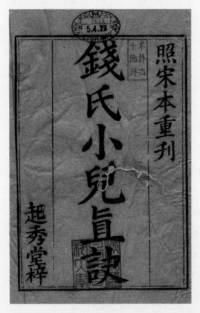

*Photoprint of Key to Therapeutics of Children's Diseases*
(Xiǎo Ér Yào Zhèng Zhí Jué，小儿药证直诀)
now preserved in the Library of CACMS

## V New Knowledge of Anatomy—*Ou Xifan's Drawing of Five Zang Organs* and *Vivid Drawings of the Body*

During the Northern Song Dynasty, ancient Chinese anatomy had a critical development. Two human anatomical activities were conducted before and after this period and two human anatomical maps—*Ou Xifan's Drawing of Five Zang Organs* and *Vivid Drawings of the Body* were produced.

During the Qingli period of Emperor Renzong of Song Dynasty (1041–1048 AD), the local government of Guangxi executed 56 rebels, including Ou Xifan, and dissected the chest and abdomen of the dead. Wu Jian (Ling Jian), the official of Yizhou, doctors and painters carefully observed the internal organs of these bodies, which were depicted by Painter Song Jing and made *Ou Xifan's Drawing of Five Zang Organs*. It is the earliest known human anatomy map. Although the map has been lost for a long time, and it is not easy to know the details, the drawing process has been recorded in many historical records and notes. Especially in the *Vivid Drawings of the Body*, there was a detailed record of this anatomical activity.

*Vivid Drawings of the Body* is an anatomical map drawn by Doctor Yang Jie and the painter during the Chongning period of Emperor Huizong of Song Dynasty (1102–1106 AD) according to the chest, abdomen, and internal organs of rebels who were executed and cut by the government. *Vivid Drawings of the Body* existed in the early Qing Dynasty, and there are written records of this map in the *Bibliography Wenyuan Pavilion* and *Mao's Collection Catalogue of Jigu Pavilion–Doctors*. Some medical books in Yuan and Ming Dynasties also transcribed their anatomical maps and explanatory texts. Although the manuscript of *Vivid Drawings of the Body* has been lost, some of its contents have been preserved by these medical books. It can be seen from the records of later medical books that the drawing of the *Vivid Drawings of the Body* is very simple, detailed and specific, which not only has the entire part of human body, like front, back, and side pictures of the human chest, abdomen, and internal organs, but also has sub-systems and sub-parts, such as the *Drawing of the Lung Side* and the right side picture of the internal chest organs; the *Drawing of Heart Qi* is a map of the relationship of primary blood vessel with lateral chest

137

and thoracic cavity; the *Drawing of the Sea of Qi and Transverse Membrane* is the morphological map of blood vessels and esophagus through which the diaphragm passes; the *Drawing of Spleen and Stomach* is the digestive system map; the *Drawing of Fenshui* draws the urinary system; the *Map of the Gate of Life, Large and Small Intestines and Bladder* draws the genitourinary system. The maps and their descriptions are consistent with the discoveries of modern anatomy.

Before the 16th century, the actual anatomy of the human body was extremely rare in Europe. The appearance and influence of *Ou Xifan's Drawing of Five Zang Organs* and *Vivid Drawings of the Body* show that the level of human anatomy in China was in the leading position in the world as early as the 11th century. Especially, *Vivid Drawings of the Body*, which has far-reaching influence in the history, is the most valuable and successful anatomical map in the Chinese ancient medical history.

# VI Song Ci and His Great Achievement of Forensic Medicine *Record for Vindication*

Since ancient times, China has attached great importance to examination, and the contents of visual inspection to examine skin wounds, flesh wounds, fractures, flesh and bone injury and so on recorded in *The Book of Rites– Proceedings of Government in the Different Months* show the germination of forensic medicine. *The Records of Doubtful Lawsuits* (951 AD), co-authored by He Ning and his son in the Five Dynasties, is the earliest existing forensic monograph in China. Since then, the anonymous *Settle A Lawsuit with Benevolence and Forgiveness* in the Song Dynasty, Zheng Ke's *Collection of Judging Lawsuits*, and Gui Wanrong's *The Washing away of Wrongs* had been published one after another, constantly enriching the research of ancient forensic medicine in China. However, most of these books are case records, which cannot be regarded as forensic examination monographs. *Record for Vindication*, written by Song Ci, can be called the first systematic forensic medicine monograph in China and in the world.

Song Ci (1186–1249 AD), courtesy-named Huifu, Han nationality, a native of Jianyang (now Nanping, Fujian Province), and a scholar, served as a senior criminal officer four times. Song Ci had been engaged in judicial and criminal prison all his life, and his long-term professional work enabled him to accumulate rich experience in forensic examination. He believed that "Death penalty is the most serious punishment in criminal cases, and the death penalty is determined by the facts of the crime, which in turn must be examined to determine". He synthesized, verified, and refined the works of corpse injury examination handed down at that time. Then, combined with his rich practical experience, he wrote *Record for Vindication* in 1247 AD. This book recorded in detail the contents of human anatomy, corpse examination, on-site examination, identification of the cause of death, and listed the symptoms of various poisons, as well as the methods of first aid and detoxification. Compared with modern forensic medicine, *Record for Vindication* not only discusses the same scope and content, but also includes the basic knowledge needed by modern forensic medicine. For example, it is of high value to wash corpses and scars with lees (distiller's grains) and vinegar in this book. It is consistent with the principle of using acid precipitation in modern forensic medicine to protect wounds, prevent external bacterial infection, reduce inflammation and fix wounds.

*Record for Vindication* involves many disciplines, such as physiology, anatomy, pathology, pharmacology, toxicology, orthopedics, surgery, and ecsomatics. It is not only a summary of forensic achievements before the Song Dynasty but also reflects the development of Chinese ancient medical science. As soon as the book was published, it immediately attracted the attention of the whole society and quickly became a necessary book for trial officials at that time. From the 13th century to the 19th century, it was used for more than 600 years, and many forensic books in later generations were also based on it. This book is not only widely circulated in China, but also very influential abroad. It has been translated into Korean, Japanese, Dutch, English, German, Russian and other languages and published overseas, making a very important contribution to the development of modern forensic medicine.

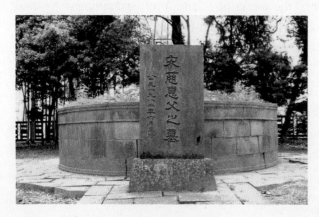

*Songci Tomb*
Located in Changmao Village, Chongluo Township, Jianyang District, Nanping City, Fujian Province

# VII The Four Famous Medical Schools in Jin and Yuan Dynasties

Before Tang and Song Dynasties, there was no academic contention in the medical field because no mature academic schools had formed. During the Jin and Yuan Dynasties, due to the exchanges and integration of medicine between Song and Liao states and various ethnic groups, as well as frequent wars, and the prevalence of folk diseases, many new problems were raised for medical research. In this context, a wide variety of schools emerged, and contention of a hundred schools of thought was formed, among which the most representative ones were Liu Wansu, Zhang Zihe, Li Dongyuan, and Zhu Danxi, who were called "Four Medical Schools in Jin and Yuan Dynasties" by later generations.

Liu Wansu (1110–1200 AD), courtesy-named Shouzhen, pseudonym named Tongxuan Chushi, and alias named Shouzhen Zi, was born in Hejian (now Hejian County, Hebei Province). He was also called Liu Hejian in later generations, and the school he founded was "Hejian School". His academic thoughts, such as "the theory of fire heat" and "the theory of movements and qi", had a significant influence on the development of Yan-Zhao medicine and had a significant influence on later generations' schools of invigorating the earth, removing the pathogen, nourishing yin and warm diseases. In the treatment method, Liu is good at using cold and cool medicines, so his school is called "Cold and Cool School". Fangfeng Tongsheng Powder, which he initiated, is a good formula for treating exterior-interior excess and clearing heat-toxin, and is still widely used in clinics.

Zhang Zihe (1156–1228 AD), a native of Henan during the Jin Dynasty, put forward the theory of "eliminating pathogenic factors to reinforce healthy qi". He believed that the pathogenic factors come from the exterior or interior and must be eliminated. If the pathogenic factors are eliminated, healthy qi will be reinforced; do not hesitate to attack pathogens, otherwise they will reside and develop over time. Zhang has unique views on the application of sweating, vomiting, and purging methods in treatment, especially pays attention to the purgative method, so he is called the representative of "Removing the Pathogen School". His academic thoughts enriched TCM's pathogenesis theory and treatment methods, and his representative work is *Confucians' Duties to their*

*Parents.*

Li Dongyuan (1180–1251 AD), also known as Li Gao, was born in Ding County, Hebei Province, and put forward the theory of "stomach qi-centeredness". It is advocated that if the spleen and stomach are healthy, it is not easy to get sick; even if it is sick, it is easy to cure. In the treatment method, he paid attention to regulating the spleen and stomach, cultivating and tonifying yuan-primordial qi, and reinforcing healthy qi to eliminate pathogenic factors, which contributes to the theory and treatment method of internal dysfunctions to the spleen and stomach. His theory significantly influenced later doctors, especially the school of warming and tonifying, and he is called the representative of "Tonifying the Spleen School" by later generations. His representative works include *Treatise on Spleen and Stomach, Clarifying Doubts about Damage from Internal and External Causes*, and so on.

Zhu Danxi (1281–1358 AD), named Zhenheng and courtesy-named Yanxiu, was born in Yiwu, Zhejiang Province, during Yuan Dynasty. He applied Neo-Confucianism thinking to medicine and the laws of nature to the human body and put forward the famous theory of "yang excess but yin insufficiency". In treatment, he paid attention to nourishing yin, which is called "Nourishing Yin School" by later generations. Zhu Danxi lived in the latest age among the four medical schools of the Jin and Yuan Dynasties. However, he absorbed the strengths of many schools and wrote *Further Discourses on the Properties of Things, Elaboration of Bureau Prescription, Danxi's Mastery of Medicine*, and so on, which played an essential role in the history of TCM.

Based on summarizing a large number of clinical practices, the four medical scientists made breakthrough innovations in the theory of TCM. Moreover, academic contention and innovation represented by them opened up new ideas, new paths, and new methods for the development of TCM, greatly enriched the treasure house of TCM theory, improved the ability of prevention and treatment of diseases by TCM, and had a profound impact on the innovation of medicine in Ming and Qing Dynasties and the later development of TCM.

## VIII Mongolian Nutritionist—Hu Sihui

Hu Sihui, a Mongolian, was born and died in an unknown year and lived in the 13th to 14th century AD. From 1314 AD to 1320 AD, he served as a palace physician of diet in the Yuan Dynasty and was responsible for the catering work at the palace. He made a study of all kinds of nutritive foods, tonic medicines, diet hygiene, and food poisoning and was a famous nutritionist in ancient times of China.

Hu Sihui compiled *Principles of Correct Diet* in the third year of Emperor Tianli (1330 AD). In the book, Hu systematically summarized and sorted out the dietetic therapy experience of the previous dynasties, inherited the dietetic therapy achievements from famous materia medica works and famous doctors of the previous generation and drew on the dietetic therapy experience in the daily life of the folk at that time. Based on the principles of preventing the disease before it arises, emphasis on diet and nourishment of the spleen and stomach, many theories and methods of diet and health care according to the health care needs of the Yuan Dynasty court and the dietary habits of aristocrats at that time are stated in *Principles of Correct Diet*. This book is divided into 3 volumes. The first volume introduces all kinds of foods and explains various taboos in the diet. The second volume deals with ingredients, diet, and dietetic therapy. The third volume is about the property and flavor, efficacy, and contraindications of rice, animals, birds, fish, fruits, vegetables, materials, and other foods. There are 230 kinds of food in total, among which 168 pictures are attached to illustrate the shapes of various foods. The book also formulates recipes with great nutritional value, highlighting the role of diet in daily health care. In addition, Hu also specifically pointed out the application objects of dietetic therapy. He paid special attention to the maternal and child dietary health, made a special discussion on the dietary taboos of women during pregnancy and lactation, and added many medicated diets that were not recorded in the previous literature. He also attached great importance to food hygiene and made many beneficial constraints on the eating habits of his time, which was very realistic dietary hygiene measures. Many of the effective remedies he listed for food poisoning are still in use today.

*Principles of Correct Diet* is a monograph that combines the food culture of Mongolian and Han nationalities. It is introduced that "the book is a collection of the exotic food, decoction, paste and herbs from various schools, prescriptions of famous doctors, and daily necessities of grains, meat, fruits, and vegetables with special flavor and benefits". From the perspective of nutrition, many viewpoints on diet and health are put forward. It is the first monograph on diet hygiene and nutrition in ancient China and the earliest in the world with high academic and historical value and is still worthy of our in-depth study and research today.

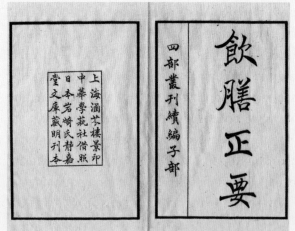

*Photoprint of Principles of Correct Diet* (Yǐn Shàn Zhèng Yào，饮膳正要) now preserved in the Library of CACMS

Chapter 5

Ming and Qing Dynasties

—Prosperity and Innovation of TCM

The Ming and Qing Dynasties are the stage of comprehensive integration and deepening development of TCM theory. The landmark achievements were the development of life gate theory, the innovation of epidemic warm disease theory, and the compilation and integration of a large number of medical books, series, and subject reference books, which greatly enriched and developed the theoretical system of TCM and made remarkable achievements. During the period of the Republic of China, slogans such as "improving TCM", "scientizing TCM", and "creating new TCM" were popular. The development of TCM showed the characteristics of convergence between Chinese and the Western medicine in this period. Although the development of TCM was not supported by the government of the Republic of China, TCM still had a deep popular base among the people and continued to develop.

# I A Masterpiece of Medical Prescription—*Prescriptions for Universal Relief*

Prescription is an essential part of the TCM system, and prescription books have been the bulk of TCM literature in the past dynasties. The development of prescription books accumulated experiential practical recipes and recorded the etiology, symptoms, and clinical treatment methods related to diseases and syndromes since the Tang and Song Dynasties. The systematic theoretical summary and prescription research began in the Song Dynasty and flourished in the Ming and Qing Dynasties. In the Ming Dynasty, the outstanding achievements of medical prescriptions should be represented by *Prescriptions for Universal Relief*, edited by Zhu Su.

*Prescriptions for Universal Relief* was written in the 23rd year of Hongwu in the Ming Dynasty (1390 AD), with a total of 426 volumes, citing various prescriptions of the past dynasties, collecting notes, miscellany, Taoist and Buddhist books, ancient and modern medical prescriptions, including pulse theory, medicinal properties, movements of qi, typhoid fever, miscellaneous diseases, gynecology, pediatrics, acupuncture, and medicinals. According to the statistics of the *Bibliography of Imperial Collection of Four Divisions*, there are 1,960 theoretical discussions, which are divided into 2,175 categories under 101 subjects, including 778 methods and 239 illustrations, and 61,739 prescriptions of doctors in the past dynasties. With a total number of tens of millions of words, under the historical conditions at that time, it could be said that it was an unprecedented innovation. This book is the giant existing prescription book in China, which is rich in collection and detailed analysis and preserves rich and precious medical prescription materials.

More than 150 kinds of prescription books are cited in *Prescriptions for Universal Relief*, and many medical books collected are now lost. *The Yongle Canon*, a large-scale book compiled in the same period, is famous for its extensiveness and variedness in content. More than 50 kinds of ancient medical books cited in *Prescriptions for Universal Relief* are not found in *The Yongle Canon*. *Bibliography of Imperial Collection of Four Divisions* evaluated this book: "It is this book that lists all the prescriptions under one syndrome, so that scholars can conform to the categories and find the answers, and comprehend the intentions of the ancients between similarities and differences. So they can compromise the uneven and irregular conditions, which is not bound by the law." Later, scholars commented on it as "a special secret technique in ancient times, which can be used for biography". The compilation of this book is of great significance for compiling lost ancient books, especially medical books of the Song and Yuan Dynasties. For today's researchers in the field of TCM, this book is also of great reference value to verify the changes in the origin and development of prescriptions and refer to similarities and differences.

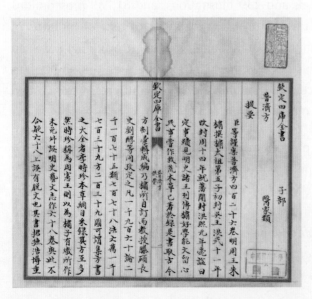

*Photoprint of Prescriptions for Universal Relief*
(Pǔ Jì Fāng，普济方 )
from *Imperial Collection of Four Divisions*
(Sì Kù Quán Shū ， 四库全书 )
in the Qing Dynasty, now preserved in the Library of CACMS

## II Vaccination against Smallpox

The first documented method of smallpox prevention by vaccination (inoculation) in China is Zhu Chungu's *Conclusion of Exanthema Variolosum*, which records that during the reign of Emperor Zhenzong of the Song Dynasty, several children of the Prime Minister Wang Dan unfortunately died of smallpox. Then he had a son named Wang Su. In order not to make Wang Su have the same disaster, Wang Dan called in many famous doctors to discuss the prevention and treatment of smallpox. He heard that there was a "magic doctor" in Emei Mountain, Sichuan Province, who could vaccinate people against smallpox, so he asked him to vaccinate Wang Su. On the 7th day after vaccination, Wang Su had fever all over his body, and after 12 days, the pox scabbed. Subsequently, the technology of inoculation against smallpox gradually became the primary method of smallpox prevention in ancient China after the continuous practice and improvement of various generations of doctors. This technology was widely popularized and spread at that time, which is inseparable from the attention of Emperor Kangxi of the Qing Dynasty.

During the Ming and Qing Dynasties, smallpox was rampant. It was recorded that many members of the Manchu royal family died of smallpox. At that time, people were afraid of smallpox as if it were a tiger, and they had no other way to avoid it when it broke out. Faced with this situation, Emperor Kangxi began to actively seek preventive measures against smallpox. In the 20th year of Kangxi's reign (1681 AD), Xu Dingbi, an assistant of the Ministry of Internal Affairs, was assigned to Jiangxi Province to look for a vaccinator, which was recommended by Li Yuegui, a local officer. After the method was proved to be effective, Zhu Chungu was introduced to inoculate the descendants of the royal family and court officials. Subsequently, Zhu Chungu served in the Imperial Hospital, where a pox division was set up to handle vaccination and treatment. After that, he was also sent to 49 banners and Kalka to vaccinate the descendants of Manchu and Mongolian officials. Emperor Kangxi once said in the *Motto of Court Training*: "In the early years, many people were afraid of smallpox. When I got the vaccination prescription, and all my children and others were vaccinated and safe from smallpox. Today, the 49 banners and the Kalka were ordered to be vaccinated. All who were inoculated recovered well." Because the emperor ordered the

149

promotion of variolation technology to prevent smallpox, "no less than 8,000 people have been vaccinated against smallpox. According to the statistics, only 20 or 30 people failed to be saved." It can be seen that this technology was relatively mature in the middle of the 18th century.

The variolation is known as the pioneer of human immunology. This technology was not only widely used in China at that time but also popularized all over the world. First it was introduced to Russia, Japan, Korea, then to Northern Europe, and Britain. It was not until 1796 when the British Jenner tried vaccinia successfully that variolation was gradually replaced by cowpox vaccination. Voltaire, a French Enlightenment thinker, once wrote in *Lettres Philosophiques*: "I heard that Chinese people had had this habit (referring to vaccination) for 100 years. This is a significant precedent and example set by a nation considered to be the most intelligent and polite in the world." It can be said that variolation technology has made great contributions to the prevention and treatment of human infectious diseases.

# III Li Shizhen and *The Grand Compendium of Materia Medica*

Li Shizhen (1518–1593 AD), courtesy-named Dongbi and art-named Binhu Shanren in his later years, was born in Qizhou, Hubei Province (now Qizhou Town, Qichun County, Hubei Province). He was born into a family of doctors and studied Confucianism since childhood. At the age of 23, he began to study medicine from his father, and his reputation as a doctor was growing day by day. At the age of 33, Li Shizhen was recommended to work in the Imperial Academy of Medicine because he cured the son of Prince Fushun, Zhu Houkun. During this period, he read many books, actively engaged in medical research, often went to the pharmacy and imperial medicine storehouses in the Imperial Academy of Medicine, carefully compared and identified medicinal materials from various places, and collected a lot of data. Combining his decades of medical experience, Li Shizhen found that there were many mistakes in ancient herbal books, so he decided to compile a new herbal book. To fulfill this grand wish, he went to Wudang Mountain, Lushan Mountain, Maoshan Mountain, Niushou Mountain, Hubei, Hunan, Anhui, Henan, and Hebei to collect medicine specimens and prescriptions. He also took fishermen, woodsmen, farmers, coachmen, pharmacists and snake catchers as his teachers, and referred to 925 kinds of books on medicine in the past dynasties. By reading extensively, he wrote tens of millions of words as notes. After 27 years and three changes in the draft, he completed *The Grand Compendium of Materia Medica*, a masterpiece of 1.92 million words in the 18th year of Wanli in the Ming Dynasty (1590 AD).

*The Grand Compendium of Materia Medica* is the greatest pharmacological works in ancient China. It is a collection of the outstanding achievements of materia medica before the Ming Dynasty, with scientific classification and rich content, which occupies a very important position in the history of world medicine. There are 1,892 medicines in *The Grand Compendium of Materia Medica*, 374 of which were added by Li Shizhen through his own interviews and investigations. In accordance with the principle of "birds of the same feather flock together, and the table of contents follows the outline", this book summarizes medicines according to their natural properties, with a total of 16 parts, which are subdivided into several categories under each part, establishing an advanced medicine classification system. The description of medicines in this book covers the name, origin, variety, form, processing method, property, taste, efficacy, and indications. The textual research of medicine varieties is scientific and rigorous, and the discussion is detailed. In addition, it also records natural science knowledge related to the forms of medicines and the ecological environment.

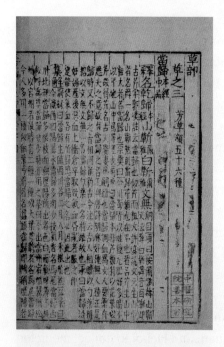

The publication of *The Grand Compendium of Materia Medica* pushed materia medica to an unprecedented height. After the late Ming Dynasty, it was published many times and had a far-reaching influence. Li Shizhen devoted his whole life to the compilation of this book. This kind of perseverance, perfect sense of responsibility and mission is also the best interpretation of traditional Chinese medicine cultural heritage for thousands of years. Up to now, Li Shizhen's thoughts on TCM and the rich contents of *The Grand Compendium of Materia Medica* still have significant guiding value for the research and development of TCM and clinical practice, and have been paid more and more attention by academia at home and abroad.

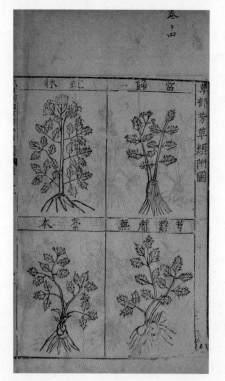

*Photoprint of The Grand Compendium of Materia Medica*
(Běn Cǎo Gāng Mù，本草纲目)
now preserved in the Library of CACMS

## IV Wu Youke's *Treatise on Pestilence* and the Innovation of Infectious Disease Theory

*Huangdi Neijing* discusses that "when five epidemics break out, both adults and children are susceptible to their infection and they all have similar symptoms", and this is the earliest documented theory of infectious disease in China. Chao Yuanfang recorded 34 syndromes of warm diseases in *General Treatise on Causes and Manifestations of All Diseases* and discussed three different types of infectious diseases, including common seasonal infectious diseases, severe infectious diseases caused by surly qi and typhoid fever. Wang Lv, a doctor in the Ming Dynasty, pointed out in the *A Discourse on Tracingback of Medical Classic*: "Warm diseases and febrile diseases are also named after the climatic condition and disease syndromes." It is pointed out that febrile disease is "hyperthermia from the inside to the outside". In the late Ming Dynasty, the theory of warm diseases gradually rose and developed, and the most representative figure was Wu Youke.

Wu Youke (1582–1652 AD), courtesy-named Youxing, a native of Wuxian County (now Suzhou, Jiangsu Province), was an epidemiologist in the late Ming and early Qing Dynasties and one of the principal founders of the ancient theory of warm diseases. According to the documents, there were 64 outbreaks of pestilence in the Ming Dynasty, and Wu experienced the plagues in Hebei, Shandong, Jiangsu, Zhejiang, and other provinces in the 14th year of Emperor Chongzhen period (1641 AD). Facing the pandemic, he voiced that "a large number of people died, not from the epidemic, but from medical treatment". Through his personal observation and clinical practice of diagnosis and application of medicines, he creatively put forward a systematic view that warm diseases are different from typhoid fever based on predecessors' discussions. In 1642 AD, he compiled and completed the *Treatise on Pestilence*, which innovated and developed the theory of infectious diseases based on traditional theories and pioneered the study of infectious diseases.

Wu also creatively put forward the "pestilential qi theory". He thought the cause of infectious diseases was "non-wind, non-cold, non-heat, and non-dampness, but there was an abnormal qi between heaven and earth, that is, pestilential qi". He also pointed out the transmission route of "pestilential qi", and held that pestilence qi "enters the human body from the nose and mouth", and whether it causes the disease is related to the amount and virulence of pestilence qi, as well as the human body's resistance. This statement scientifically foresees the transmission route of infectious diseases. At the same time, based on many practical identification experience, Wu pointed out that people and livestock would get sick because of pestilence qi. However, different types of pestilence qi can cause different diseases. "Everything has its desirability and contraindications, and those who are desirable benefit and those who are contraindicated lose, and those who lose also restrain, so all things have their own restraint." It can be seen that he has a scientific understanding of the specificity of infectious disease pathogens.

After the book was written, *Treatise on Pestilence* was circulated widely and had a far-reaching influence. At that time, there was no microscope to observe pathogenic microorganisms such as bacteria and viruses, Wu had scientifically foreseen their existence and made an in-depth and systematic discussion on the etiology and transmission routes of warm diseases and made significant contributions to the systematization of warm diseases theory.

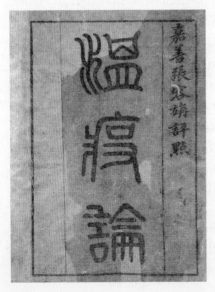

*Photoprint of Treatise on Pestilence*
(Wēn Yì Lùn，温疫论)
now preserved in the Library of CACMS

## V Chen Shigong and *Orthodox Manual of External Diseases*

Chen Shigong (1555–1636 AD), courtesy-named Yuren and art-named Ruoxu, a native of Nantong, Jiangsu Province, was a famous surgeon in Ming Dynasty. He studied surgery since childhood. He learned from Li Lunming, a famous writer and medical scientist, and was deeply influenced by his teacher. "The internal disease may not relate to the external disease, while the external disease must be rooted in the interior," Li Lunming believed, which became the motto of Chen Shigong's decades-long surgical career. He inherited and developed Li Lunming's viewpoint, advocating that surgical diseases should be treated internally or by combining internal treatment with external treatment, emphasizing the combination of external surgery and oral-taking medicine.

In 1617 AD, Chen Shigong compiled and completed the book *Orthodox Manual of External Diseases*, which consists of 12 volumes and 157 articles. For diseases, such as carbuncle and abscess, deep-rooted sore (hard furuncle), multiple deep abscess, cervical scrofula, gall, intestinal abscess, hemorrhoids, vitiligo, scald, scabies, injuries, skin and ENT diseases, were classified. "Classify the categories clearly, generalize them with theories, relate them with songs, and explain them with law and theory, so that even very small scabies will not be missed." More than 100 common surgical diseases are systematically discussed in the book, and the etiology, pathology, symptoms, syndromes, diagnosis, and treatment methods of each kind of disease are discussed. In the treatment method, Chen advocated a combination of internal and external approaches, "elimination", "support" and "tonification" and both oral-taking medicine and external treatment methods. He inherited and developed toe amputation, pharyngeal foreign body removal, mandibular dislocation reduction, and tracheal suture in surgical treatment. In addition, he also designed and manufactured many simple and effective surgical instruments, such as creating oolong needles for foreign body removal from the pharynx and removing nasal polyps with fine copper chopsticks. These were of great significance to the surgical level at that time. *Orthodox Manual of External Diseases* also discussed skin diseases and tumors. For tumors, Chen believed that a tumor could be treated and cured if it was detected early and its source was identified.

The *Orthodox Manual of External Diseases* is famous for its detailed analysis and incisive treatment, which reflects the important achievements of surgery in China before Ming Dynasty. It is the classic works of TCM surgery. After publication, it was widely circulated and spread to Japan and other countries, which has high academic value.

# VI Outstanding Achievements of Ophthalmology Monograph *Essence on the Silvery Sea*

*Essence on the Silvery Sea* is a well-known ophthalmic work both at home and abroad. Sun Simiao of Tang Dynasty compiled the current edition. Most scholars today think that it was written under his name, while most domestic scholars think it was written in Ming Dynasty. Taoism regards the eye as the silver sea, so *Essence on the Silvery Sea* means that this book is rich in the subtle essence of ophthalmic principles, prescriptions, and medicines. Based on the achievements of ophthalmology in the previous dynasties, this book supplements various diagnosis and treatment methods for eye diseases and closely combines ophthalmic theory with medicine and surgical treatment, which has high academic value.

The two-volume *Essence on the Silvery Sea* contains 82 diseases, mainly including eyelid generating wind millet (trachoma), hyperopia, and myopia, of which 80 symptoms are illustrated with pictures to mark the lesion sites or pathological conditions. The description of ophthalmic surgery methods in the book is quite detailed. There are clear records of surgical methods, such as scraping-washing, hooking, cutting, needling, and cauterizing, surgical procedures, indications, and contraindications. The treatment difficulty and different treatment effects of ophthalmic diseases caused by different reasons are also involved. For example, for hyphema and vitreous hemorrhage caused by diseases of liver and kidney meridians, it is emphasized that "This blood is difficult to eliminate". For hyphema and vitreous hemorrhage caused by external injury, it is pointed out that "Blood perfusion in the pupils caused by trauma or surgical errors will quickly subside". Some of these surgical and external treatments recorded in the book are also commonly used in modern Western medicine. In addition, *Essence on the Silvery Sea* also makes an essential contribution to the diagnosis of ophthalmic diseases, pointing out that "When observing the eyes, we should first inspect the spirit of the pupil, secondly the wind wheel, thirdly the white of the eyes, finally the eyelid, which are the key points of ophthalmology".

*Essence on the Silvery Sea* is meticulous in syndrome differentiation, rich in texts and pictures, fair and unbiased in method establishment, and practical and influential in the prescription selection, which has a far-reaching influence on the development of ophthalmology in the Ming Dynasty and later. *Bibliography of Imperial Collection of Four Divisions* in the Qing Dynasty commented on it: "It is quite clear to differentiate and analyze various syndromes. Its methods are combined with tonifying and purging, cold and warm [medicinals] are used together, and there is no disadvantage of being partial to the main one." The discussion in the book on the treatment prescriptions for ophthalmic diseases, the method of removing cataracts with metal needles, the prescriptions, and the properties of commonly used medicinals in ophthalmology still play an essential role in the clinical practice of ophthalmology of TCM. The book has also been translated into English by Western scholars and is extensively spread worldwide.

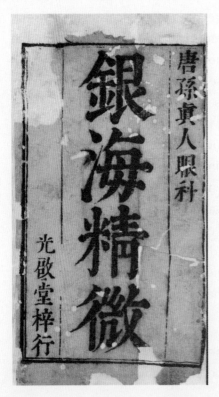

*Photoprint of Essence on the Silvery Sea*
(Yín Hǎi Jīng Wēi, 银海精微)
now preserved in the Library of CACMS

## VII *The Grand Compendium of Acupuncture and Moxibustion*: Serving as A Link between Past and Future

*The Grand Compendium of Acupuncture and Moxibustion* is a work of acupuncture and moxibustion, which was written by Yang Jizhou in the Ming Dynasty and re-edited by Jin Xian. It was first published in the 29th year of Wanli in the Ming Dynasty (1601 AD), with 10 volumes.

Yang Jizhou, named Jishi, was born in Sanqu (now Liuduyang Village, Quzhou City, Zhejiang Province) during the Ming Dynasty. The Yang family had been doctors for generations, and his grandfather used to be an imperial doctor at the Imperial Academy of Medicine, who was quite prestigious. Yang Jizhou read many books when he was young and then abandoned Confucianism to become a doctor. He never stopped studying medicine. Because he felt that "All the books from different schools will not be collected in one book", he comprehensively referenced the main idea of the medical works handed down from the older generations of his family and the discussion of acupuncture and moxibustion from different schools' medical works, collected the same and examined the differences, and compiled them into *Secrets of Hygienic Acupuncture and Moxibustion*. But this book was not published. It happened that Zhao Wenbing, the supervisory censor of Shanxi Province, suffered from flaccidity and arthralgia. He had been treated in many ways, but did not respond well to the treatments. Yang Jizhou was invited to Shanxi for diagnosis and treatment. Zhao Wenbing only received three needles, and flaccidity and arthralgia were cured on the spot. To appreciate Yang Jizhou, Zhao Wenbing decided to help him print the book *Secrets of Hygienic Acupuncture and Moxibustion* and entrusted Jin Xian, a native of Jinyang, to revise the anthology. However, Yang Jizhou believed that the manuscript's contents were still defective. Therefore, based on the *Secrets of Hygienic Acupuncture and Moxibustion* and combined with more than 40 years of clinical experience, more than 20 crucial acupuncture works before the Ming Dynasty were compiled, such as *Compilation of Medical Classics, Compilation of Acupuncture and Moxibustion, Classic of Acupuncture and Moxibustion, Introduction to Traditional Chinese Medicine* and *Medical Complete Book of Ancient and Modern*. He finally finished the complete and practical monograph *The Grand Compendium of Acupuncture and Moxibustion*.

This book is rich in content, extensively recording the discussions on acupuncture and moxibustion in ancient medical books, such as *Huangdi Neijing* and *Classic of Questioning*. It also included acupuncture songs and poems compiled by famous doctors in the past dynasties. Besides, Yang re-researched acupoints, meridians, and acupuncture operation techniques in the past dynasties, and recorded points combination, prescriptions and treatment cases of various diseases and syndromes. This book comprehensively presents the development of acupuncture and moxibustion before the Ming Dynasty with systematic and complete theories of acupuncture and moxibustion, integrating the clinical experience of many acupuncture practitioners. It is considered as the third major summary in the history of acupuncture and moxibustion after *Neijing* and *A-B Classic of Acupuncture and Moxibustion*. Since its publication in the Wanli period of the Ming Dynasty, this book has been translated into English, Japanese, German, French, Latin, and other languages. There are still 47 versions, with a new version published every 6.8 years on average. The number of its publications, its wide spread, the great influence, and the long reputation are all rare in history. The publication of *The Grand Compendium of Acupuncture and Moxibustion* indicated that acupuncture and moxibustion in ancient China reached a quite mature stage. Most later generations regard *The Grand Compendium of Acupuncture and Moxibustion* as one of the most important reference books, which plays an essential role in connecting the past with the future in the development history of acupuncture and moxibustion.

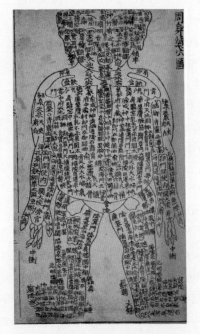

*The figure of total acupoints in the whole body contained in The Grand Compendium of Acupuncture and Moxibustion* (Zhēn Jiǔ Dà Chéng, 针灸大成 ) now preserved in the Library of CACMS

# VIII A Great Master in Warm Disease Theory—Ye Tianshi

Ye Tianshi (1667–1746 AD), given-name Gui, courtesy-named Tianshi, and art-named Xiangyan, was born in Wuxian County, Jiangsu Province (now Suzhou, Jiangsu Province). He was a famous medical scientist in the Qing Dynasty, specializing in treating seasonal epidemic diseases, measles, and smallpox, and was the first doctor to discover scarlet fever in China. His achievements in warm diseases are particularly outstanding, as he pioneered the syndrome differentiation outline of "wei-defense, qi, ying-nutrient, and blood" for warm diseases. He was one of the founders of warm diseases and established a new way for warm disease treatment based on syndrome differentiation.

Ye Tianshi was born into a medical family. His grandfather and father both worked as doctors. When he was young, he was influenced and taught by his family members. When he was 14 years old, his father died, and he learned from his father's disciple, Zhu. In the following 10 years, he learned from 17 teachers successively. "Hearing that someone is good at treating a certain syndrome, he immediately went and learn from the doctor with a respectful attitude." He had a high reputation among the people because of his drawing on the strength of every school, his assiduous study, thorough understanding, and remarkable therapeutic effects in the treatment. He was too busy diagnosing and treating diseases to write books all his life. These books, such as *Treatise on Epidemic Febrile Diseases*, *Guide to Clinical Practice with Medical Records*, *Ye Tianshi's Medical Case*, and *Unrecorded Medical Record of Ye Tianshi*, were all compiled and edited by his disciples according to his dictation or notes in clinical practice.

Ye first distinguished typhoid fever from warm diseases in terms of etiology, sensory pathway, and transmission law and pointed out clearly that "heat pathogen" is the leading cause of warm diseases. Secondly, he put forward the doctrine of "upper attack of heat pathogen firstly to the lung and then adverse transmission to the pericardium (the mechanism of the onset of most acute warm diseases starting from the upper respiratory tract, and the heat pathogen first invades the lung and the superficial defensive system and then results in the absence of consciousness even worse)", which summarizes the development and transmission of warm diseases and becomes the general outline of understanding exogenous warm diseases. According to the development of warm diseases pathology, the dialectical method of defending qi and nourishing blood was established, and the law of transmission and change of warm diseases was pointed out, that is, "Generally speaking, qi is after wei-defence, blood is after ying-nutrient." It can be summarized into four stages: wei-defence, qi, ying-nutrient and blood, and "the method of sweating can be used when the pathogen enters wei-defence, and it is appropriate to clear qi when the pathogen enters qi. When the pathogen enters ying-nutrient, it can still clear heat in the ying-nutrient phase, and when the pathogen enters the blood, cooling blood and dissipating blood are needed". The treatment principles were summarized. Ye also detailed the significance of tongue examination, tooth examination, and macula discrimination in diagnosing warm diseases, contributing to the clinical diagnosis of warm diseases.

In his life, Ye trained many famous doctors and left a large number of medical records for later generations to read. "Speaking of medicine, Ye Gui is regarded as the master all over the north and south. For more than 100 years, Ye Gui has had the most private disciples," the *Qing History Draft* recorded. Ye lived for 80 years and always kept in awe of medicine. Before he died, he warned his descendants, "As for the dos and don'ts in medicine, you must be gifted and sensitive, and read thousands of books, and then you can use your skills to help the world. Otherwise, there are few who do not kill people. They use medicine as their knives. When I die, posterity will have to be very careful about talking about medicine."

# IX Wu Jvtong and *Detailed Analysis of Epidemic Warm Diseases*

Wu Jvtong (1758–1836 AD), given-name Tang, courtesy-named Peiheng, and art-named Jvtong, was born in Shanyang County, Huai'an (now Huai'an District, Huai'an City, Jiangsu Province) in the Qing Dynasty. *Detailed Analysis of Epidemic Warm Diseases* is his masterpiece. He is an important representative of the school of warm diseases after Ye Tianshi and Xue Xue.

Wu Jvtong was born into a scholarly family. Influenced by his father, Wu studied Confucianism since childhood, hoping to win academic honors in imperial examinations. However, when he was 19 years old, his father passed away after a long illness. After reading "People only pursue fame and fortune—these external things, but forget their own health and life" in the preface of Zhang Zhongjing's *Treatise on Cold Pathogenic Disease*, Wu gave up obtaining academic honor and devoted himself to saving people and helping the society. He experienced many epidemics in his life, and his relatives also died of warm diseases, so he devoted himself to studying warm diseases. He thought that although Wu Youke's *Treatise on Pestilence* was very broad in discussion and presented what had never been presented before, but it was somewhat fragmented and complicated to scrutinize its presentation. Ye Tianshi held moderate theory and elaborate establishment of methods, but there were medical cases scattered among miscellaneous diseases, and many people overlooked and did not delve into them. Therefore, he devoted himself to research and combined his clinical experience with textual research on *Huangdi Neijing*, *Treatise on Febrile Diseases*, and other books. Combined with the understanding of warm diseases by doctors of all ages, he wrote *Detailed Analysis of Epidemic Warm Diseases*. This book marks the formation of a complete theoretical system of warm diseases of TCM and is an essential milestone in the history of the development of TCM. Today, it still has essential reference value in the prevention and treatment of warm diseases.

Wu Jvtong fundamentally differentiated typhoid fever from warm diseases. The origin of typhoid fever lies in water; the origin of warm diseases lies in the fire. He considered typhoid fever and warm diseases are different like water to fire. Secondly, warm diseases were divided into nine types: wind warm,

warm heat, epidemic febrile diseases, warm toxin, summer heat, damp warm, autumn dryness, winter warmth, and warm malaria. Epidemic febrile diseases are only one of the nine kinds of warm diseases, which are highly infectious. In comparison, the other eight kinds can be distinguished from seasons and disease manifestations, thus determining the research scope of the theory of warm diseases. In the pathogenesis of warm diseases, Wu Jvtong thought it changed from sanjiao. He related the transmission of warm diseases with the pathogenesis of zang-fu viscera, and he said, "Warm diseases enter from nose and mouth, nasal qi passes through the lung, mouth qi passes through the stomach, and lung diseases will reversely transmit to the pericardium. If the upper jiao disease is not treated, the pathogen will pass to the stomach and spleen of the middle jiao. If the middle jiao disease is not treated, the pathogen will pass to the liver and kidney of the lower jiao. It begins at the upper jiao, and ends in the lower jiao." It supplemented and perfected Ye Tianshi's syndrome differentiation of wei-defense, qi, ying-nutrient, and blood. In the book, Wu Jvtong also established the primary method of clearing heat and nourishing yin and put forward the treatment prescriptions for different stages of warm diseases: using Yinqiao Powder and Sangju Drink in wei-defense; using Baihu Decoction and Chengqi Decoction in qi; using Qingying Decoction and Qinggong Decoction in ying-nutrient; using Xijiao Dihuang Decoction in blood. Wu Jvtong significantly improved the theory, method, prescription, and medical system for warm diseases.

# X The Most Authoritative Textbook on TCM—*Golden Mirror of the Medical Tradition*

In the early Qing Dynasty, the social economy developed rapidly, the national strength flourished, and Palace medicine peaked. In 1739 AD, Emperor Qianlong ordered Wu Qian, a famous doctor in the Imperial Academy of Medicine, to preside over the compilation of a large set of medical books to promote the cultural governance "to get medicine on the right track", "let the teacher follow this book to teach; students learn from it".

Wu Qian, courtesy-named Liuji, was born in She County, Anhui Province. Later generations called him, Yu Chang and Zhang Lu the three great masters in the early Qing Dynasty. After receiving imperial orders, to correct the problems existing in medical classics and various medical books, such as "difficult words, wrong transmission and writing, or extensive but shallow knowledge, or miscellaneous but not uniform". He not only referred to the internal library collection of the imperial court but also ordered the collection of all kinds of old and new medical books and experience prescriptions from all over the country. He also selected more than 70 officials who were proficient in medicine, liberal arts, and sciences to compile them together. They sorted out the miscellany, selected the essence, and learned from others. It took 3 years to complete the editing, and Emperor Qianlong gave it the title *Golden Mirror of Medicine*. Since 1749, the Imperial Academy of Medicine of the Qing Dynasty had designated the *Golden Mirror of Medicine* as a textbook for medical students, which had gradually become a national medical teaching standard and had been implemented throughout the state with far-reaching influence.

*Golden Mirror of the Medical Tradition* is a series of medical books of teaching and clinical diagnosis and treatment. It pays attention to practicality and explains profound theories in simple language. The book consists of 90 volumes and 15 fascicles. The content is extremely rich, collecting the essence of the famous works in the past dynasties from the Spring and Autumn Period and the Warring States Period to the Ming and Qing Dynasties. It included 17 volumes of *Treatise on Cold Pathogenic Disease*, 8 volumes of the *Synopsis of Golden Chamber*, 8 volumes of famous medical prescriptions, 1 volume of four diagnostic methods, 1 volume of five evolutive phases and six climatic factors, 3 volumes of typhoid fever's mastery, 5 volumes of miscellaneous disease methods, 6 volumes of gynecological methods, 6 volumes of pediatrics methods, 4 volumes of variola methods, 1 volume of vaccination methods, 16 volumes of surgical methods, 2 volumes of ophthalmology methods, 8 volumes of acupuncture and moxibustion methods, and 4 volumes of bonesetting methods, with a total of about 1.6 million words. This book not only collected many ancient prescriptions but also revised the famous doctor Zhang Zhongjing's works *Treatise on Cold Pathogenic Disease* and *Synopsis of Golden Chamber*. Its purpose was to "make people who work as doctors are not mistaken by common saying, and know that Zhongjing can treat both typhoid fever and miscellaneous diseases, as make the two books exist together in the world". This book is one of the most perfect and concise comprehensive TCM book in China, which has pictures, texts, prescriptions, and theories and is suitable for beginners and can be used as reference for doctors in the clinical diagnosis and treatment of diseases. It is the first popular medical series with the property of teaching materials in China.

The *Golden Mirror of the Medical Tradition* has apparent characteristics of the epochal character with a detailed reading. It adapted to the disease spectrum of China in the 18th century, especially suited the clinical practice, effectively improved the harm of the smallpox epidemic at that time, and set up a special variola department, which made the theory and technique integrated and upgraded, and was widely used. This book was later included in *Imperial Collection of Four Divisions*. It is highly evaluated by the *Bibliography of Imperial Collection of Four Divisions*.

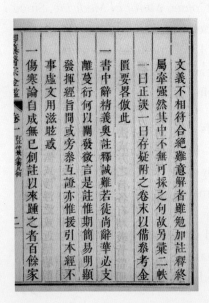

*Photoprint of Golden Mirror of the Medical Tradition* (Yī Zōng Jīn Jiàn，医宗金鉴) now preserved in the Library of CACMS

# XI The Great Master of External Treatment—Wu Shangxian

Wu Shangxian (1806–1886 AD), given-name Zun, formerly known as An'ye, courtesy-named Shangxian, Shiji or Quanxian, and art-named Qianyu Jvshi or Qianyu Laoren, was born in Qiantang (now Hangzhou) and was a famous medical scientist in the Qing Dynasty. Wu was born into a literary family and studied Confucianism since childhood. His family influenced him, and he read all the subsets of classics and history. In the 14th year of Daoguang (1834 AD), he was admitted to the First-degree Scholar (a successful candidate in the imperial examinations at the provincial level). He became a post-magistrate of a county, and the highest position was Cabinet Secretary in Inner Court. Later, due to illness, he did not participate in the capital-level examination. Since then, he gradually lost interest in his official career and fame and followed his father to "live in Yangzhou, study as a doctor besides poetry and prose". From then on, he determined to be a good doctor. He studied medicine hard, reading broadly, including *Miraculous Pivot, Plain Questions, Treatise on Cold Pathogenic Disease, Synopsis of Golden Chamber*, and other famous medical books of the past dynasties.

In 1851 AD, the Taiping Rebellion broke out and soon spread to the whole Yangtze River Delta in the south. Wu and his family took refuge in Taizhou to avoid the war, where they saved people using external treatment. Due to the war and humid local climate, farmers waded and cultivated, which resulted in a high incidence of bi syndrome. Besides, diseases such as schistosomiasis were also prevalent. People could not get timely and effective medical treatment due to the limitation of economic and medical conditions, resulting in a large number of deaths. At that time, other medicines were scarce. To treat patients, Wu extensively learned from predecessors' experience and created a method of treating external diseases for internal diseases, such as treating internal and external diseases, pediatric and gynecologocal diseases with plasters, fumigation, and washing methods. These were simple, effective, and widely applicable, so they were trendy among the general public. In the third year of Tongzhi (1864 AD), he absorbed the external treatment from predecessors and ancient books, collected folk external treatment methods, and wrote the first monograph on external treatment methods in Chinese history, *Rhymed Discourse for Topical Remedies* (also known as *Treatment Medicine Theory*). This book comprehensively and systematically sorted out and summarized the external treatment methods of TCM, discussed the treatment mechanism of plaster in detail, and pointed out the preparation and application methods of plaster. Wu lived in a significant era of "Western learning introduced into China", and Westen medicine gradually spread to China. However, Wu did not blindly exclude foreigners but absorbed the strengths of Western external treatment based on insisting on TCM. This book also introduces the external treatment methods of Western medicine, such as vomiting blood and epistaxis, and the blood transfusion method. In addition, he also absorbed some medical treatments for ethnic minorities, such as Jianyang Pills (Huichun Dan), a Mongolian secret recipe for treating yin syndrome with cold damage. Its rich content and unique insights open up a broad way for later generations to explore external treatment. It is worthy of modern medical application and in-depth study.

Wu was neither confined to the ancient nor to the outside world. He was good at learning and was a pioneering medical scientist. Because of his outstanding contribution to the external treatment of TCM, Wu was honored as the "master of external treatment".

# XII Ding's Family of Menghe Medical School and Modern TCM Education

Menghe Medical School originated in 1626 AD, and it is one of the best preserved TCM families with complete subjects and the most significant number of heirs after direct line. Menghe Medical School is famous for four families of Fei, Ma, Chao, and Ding, and the representative of Ding's family is Mr. Ding Ganren. Although he became famous late, he was a master of Menghe Medical School.

Ding Ganren, given-name Zezhou, is a native of Menghe Town, Changzhou City. There were many famous doctors in Menghe Town, among which Ma Peizhi, Fei Boxiong, and Chao Chongshan were the most famous. Three generations of Ding's family were doctors, and his cousin Ding Songxi studied medicine from Fei Boxiong, the founder of Menghe Medical School. Ding Ganren was sickly since childhood and had an indissoluble bond with TCM decoction. He first learned from Ding Songxi in Menghe, then studied medicine from Ma Shaocheng in Yvtang, studied surgery from Chao Chongshan, and later learned from Wang Lianshi, a famous typhoid fever doctor in Anhui Province. In his later years, he studied the theories of Four Medical Schools of the Jin and Yuan Dynasties, Wu Youke, Ye Tianshi, and Wang Mengying, and learned from others. He respected Zhang Zhongjing in clinical diagnosis, characterized by disease differentiation, flexible medication, internal and external participation, and exterior and interior.

In the late Qing Dynasty and the early Republic of China, a group of people with lofty ideals, objectively analyzed the advantages of Chinese and Western medicine represented by Mr. Ding Ganren of Menghe Medical School. They advocated the integration of Chinese and Western medicine and the modernization of TCM, and set up the banner of defending and revitalizing national medical culture. Mr. Ding took the promotion of TCM as his duty, determined to establish schools, trained successors, and united with fellow scholars Xia Yingtang and Xie Guan to raise funds to establish schools. In 1916 AD, he creatively combined thousands of years of TCM teachers with the education mode of Western colleges and universities. He founded the "Shanghai Special School of TCM" (now Shanghai University of TCM), which was officially opened in July 1917 AD, creating a precedent for modern TCM education. Then, two Guangyi TCM Hospitals in southern and northern Shanghai were set up successively to provide clinical practice bases for students. After two years, the "Women's Special School of TCM" was founded. He wrote *Compilation of Pulse Classic*, *Compilation of TCM Medical Classics*, and *Compilation of Medicine Property*, all of which were textbooks of the Shanghai Special School of TCM in the early years. Required courses in Western medicine, such as physiological anatomy and pathology, had been set up to absorb Western medical knowledge. Students had been organized to study at Guangyi TCM Hospital in southern and northern Shanghai to combine theory with practice closely. This brought up many high-level TCM talents, such as Cheng Menxue and Huang Wendong, who served as presidents of the Shanghai College of TCM after the founding of the People's Republic of China. Ding Jiwan, Cao Zhongheng, Liu Zuotong, Wang Yiren, Sheng Mengxian, Zhang Boyu, and Qin Bowei were top students who graduated from Shanghai Special School of TCM in the early days. It can be said that "its medical reputation is all over the sea, and plums are all over the world".

Mr. Ding Ganren founded the first TCM school in modern China, pioneered the education of modern TCM, and changed the single way of training TCM teachers to inherit from their families. Undoubtedly, his pioneering work made great contribution to the development of modern TCM, so it has been forever recorded in history.

# XIII The First Comprehensive Dictionary of TCM—*Grand Dictionary of Chinese Medicine*

*Grand Dictionary of Chinese Medicine* (*Dictionary* for short) was compiled by Mr. Xie Guan and his disciples and was completed in 1921 AD. It is the first comprehensive dictionary of TCM in China, which has a far-reaching influence and is still a necessary reference book for medical history researchers.

In his later years, the author Xie Guan, courtesy-named Liheng and art-named Chengzhai Laoren was born in Wujin, Jiangsu Province. His uncle, Xie Lansheng and Xie Baochu, are famous doctors in Menghe Town, and his father, Xie Zhongying, is a great geographer. Therefore, Xie Guan read the geography books collected at home since childhood and recited *Huangdi Neijing*, *Classic of Questioning*, *Treatise on Cold Pathogenic Disease*, *Synopsis of Golden Chamber*, and materia medica classics. Xie Guan studied at Soochow University in Suzhou. In 1905 AD, he went to the Guangdong University of Law and Politics to teach geography for three years. After returning to Shanghai, he became the president of Chengzhong School. Subsequently, Xie Guan worked in The Commercial Press in Shanghai twice. Since the late Qing Dynasty, Western medicine spread eastward, and the dispute between Chinese and Western medicine had never stopped, and Shanghai at that time was the central battlefield of the dispute. Xie Guan believed that TCM is bright and brilliant, and ancient and modern medical books are abundant, which are difficult to understand because they are profound, or they are not correct. Therefore, there were many medical students but few generalists, which led to the misunderstanding of TCM. So when Xie Guan was the president of Shanghai Shenzhou University of TCM, he began to compile the *Dictionary* at the request of the TCM community and The Commercial Press. Xie led 12 people to work hard day and night, and expanded it into the *Dictionary* based on the theory system of the past dynasties.

The *Dictionary* includes 7 categories: disease name, medicine name, prescription name, body, doctor, medical book, and medicine, with more than 37,000 entries and about 3.5 million words. The arrangement method takes the stroke of the first character as the order, and those with the same first character take the stroke of the second character as the order. For the convenience of retrieval, there are also term index and heading index. At that time, the *Dictionary* contained two distinct characteristics: First, it collected a wide range of books. Xie wrote in the preface: "The lost books in Korea and Japan are collected." Second, there is a vast number of books collected. In the introduction, Xie said, "There are only over 100 kinds of medical books recorded in *Complete Library in the Four Branches of Literature*. This book collects old books involving the works of Koreans and Japanese. It is a summary of more than 2,000 kinds, which serves as a ladder for textual research on ancient and modern medical books." The *Dictionary* was revised and republished in July 1926 and again in August 1933, marked as "the first edition after the national disaster". After the founding the People's Republic of China, the Commercial Press reprinted and distributed the *Dictionary* three times in December 1954, April 1955, and August 1955 to cooperate with the central government to implement the Party's TCM policies, which made the *Dictionary* spread all over the country and even overseas. Needless to say, there are some mistakes in the annotation of the *Dictionary*. If measured by the current dictionary format guidelines, there are also some shortcomings. However, the defects cannot obscure the splendor of the jade. It is still an important reference book for benefiting the medical circles and enlightening the scholars of younger age, and it shines brilliantly in the long history of TCM.

# XIV The Pioneer of Integrated Chinese and Western Medicine— Zhang Xichun

Zhang Xichun (1860–1933 AD), courtesy-named Shoufu, born in Zhucheng, Shandong Province, a native of Yanshan County, Hebei Province, is one of the representative figures of the Huitong School of Chinese and Western Medicine and a leading medical scholar in modern TCM and is praised by later generations as "the hero of Xuanqi and the model of medical circles". In 1893 AD, after Zhang Xichun failed again in the imperial examination for the second time, he taught medicine while studying as instructed by his father. In 1911 AD, Zhang Xichun became a military doctor and began his professional medical career. In 1916 AD, Lida TCM Hospital, the first TCM hospital in Shenyang, was founded and he served as the dean. His *Records of Traditional Chinese and Western Medicine in Combination* is "a must-read book for doctors".

He devoted himself to the academic thought of TCM concerning Western medicine and complemented each other's advantages. Western learning spread to the East in the late Qing Dynasty and the early Republic of China. Zhang Xichun devoted himself to the communication between Chinese and Western medicine and advocated taking TCM as the main body, taking the strengths of Western medicine and making up for the weaknesses of TCM. He advocated, "If we want our medicine to reach its peak, we must communicate with Chinese and Western medicine." He believed that "Chinese and Western physiology should be adopted, and philosophers should be involved in talking about physiology, and then they should be integrated with their ideas. Physiology revealed the principle of keeping in good health; the principle of keeping in good health is clear, and the principle of treating diseases is clear". Zhang Xichun actively sought the commonalities between TCM and Western medicine from physiology, pathology, and pharmacology. By comparison, he concluded that "there are differences between Chinese and Western theories on medicinal properties, but they are similar in root".

Zhang Xichun advocated new theories and practiced diligently. He respected the ancient rather than sticking to it, dared to innovate, and did not learn from the old paper. He advocated, "If you read the method of *Huangdi Neijing* and study carefully what it is credible, you can open the door of infinite methods. Those untrustworthy places may have been written by later generations in the name of Yellow Emperor, so it was left undiscussed." In addition, Zhang Xichun believed that "If you do not go through anything in the world and pay attention to it from time to time, you cannot say it exactly". Therefore, in order to verify the curative effect of the syndrome, he once chewed one or two qian of Gansui, purged much water, and coagulable phlegm, and realized that Gansui had the function of transforming stubborn phlegm. Moreover, he chewed 30 grains of pricklyash, knowing it had toxic side effects. He had repeatedly confirmed and deepened his clinical experience and wrote more than 160 prescriptions by himself, known as the "master of medical experimental school".

Zhang Xichun had a rigorous scholarship and had pupils everywhere. In addition to studying medicine diligently, Zhang Xichun settled in Tianjin in 1928 AD, founded the Correspondence School of TCM, and set up the "Chinese-Western Huitong Medical Society" to train successors. Disciples such as Zhou Yuxi in Longchang, Chen Aitang and Li Weinong in Rugao, Sun Yuquan and Li Baohe in Tianjin, and Zhong Xiaoqiu in Liaoning are all famous doctors.

Zhang Xichun's academic principle of "referring to Western medicine theories, focusing on the academic thought of TCM", is the herald of the modern integration of Chinese and Western medicine. Taking the strengths of Western medicine for my use, breaking through the old theory inherited by predecessors, abandoning the habit of worshiping the ancient, and accepting experimental scientific thought are still worthy of reference and learning by every TCM practitioner.

Chapter 6

Rebirth and Brilliance of TCM

Since the founding of the People's Republic of China, the Party and the government have attached great importance to the development of TCM and issued a series of principles and policies. The Party and the government always adhere to the equal emphasis on TCM and Western medicine (WM) and strive to create a medical and health service system and a health development model with Chinese characteristics in which TCM and WM complement each other and develop in a coordinated manner. TCM has made fruitful achievements in medical treatment, health care, scientific research, education, industry, and culture. At present, the voice and influence of TCM in the field of international traditional medicine continues to rise. TCM has spread to 196 countries and regions and has become an important area of cooperation between China and Association of Southeast Asian Nations (ASEAN), the European Uinon (EU), the African Union (AU), Latin American Community and Caribbean States, the Shanghai Cooperation Organization, BRICS, and other regions and mechanisms. TCM, which embodies the wisdom of the Chinese nation for thousands of years, is setting sail in the historical coordinates of the new era and will surely make more significant contributions to the construction of a healthy China and the wellbeing of mankind.

# I Chairman Mao Zedong's Great Attention on TCM

At the beginning of the founding of the People's Republic of China (PRC), there were many epidemics and a shortage of medical care and medicines. The medical and health conditions were very backward, and the national health situation was very severe. At that time, there were only over 20,000 WM doctors in our country, and although there were hundreds of thousands of TCM doctors in China, they could not function properly. Faced with this situation, Chairman Mao Zedong put forward a series of essential thoughts on developing TCM. In 1949, Chairman Mao Zedong stressed the direction of TCM during an audience with representatives of national health administrators. From the perspective of protecting and developing TCM, he emphatically pointed out that only by uniting TCM well, improving TCM, and doing its work well can it shoulder the arduous task of health work for hundreds of millions of people.

Chairman Mao Zedong spoke highly of the practical value of TCM many times. He pointed out that "TCM is a great treasure house, which should be explored and improved". He not only put forward some measures to promote the development of TCM from a macro perspective but also pointed out the development path of TCM and, at the same time, gave specific guidance to the practice of TCM in the PRC. In the 1950s, Chairman Mao Zedong gave guidance on TCM almost every year to correctly implement the principles and policies towards TCM. He emphasized that all provinces and cities with good conditions should offer TCM classes to WM doctors to study, which was expected to last for two years. In 1954, Chairman Mao Zedong gave essential instructions on the issue of TCM and ancient TCM books, pointing out that TCM should be well-protected and developed. TCM in our country has a history of thousands of years and is a highly precious wealth of the motherland. If it is allowed to decline, it will be our fault. TCM books should be sorted out. Knowledgeable TCM doctors should be organized to first translate some useful ancient texts into modern texts in a planned and focused way. When the time is ripe, they should be organized to compile a set of systematic TCM books based on their own experience.

In the period after PRC's founding, TCM's development encountered some delays and difficulties. There were some cases of contempt, discrimination, and rejection of TCM. For example, the public medical system did not reimburse the cost of TCM, large hospitals did not recruit TCM doctors, TCM continuing education schools encouraged TCM practitioners to switch to WM, medical colleges and universities did not offer TCM courses, and some articles even openly claimed that TCM was "feudal medicine", advocating the elimination of TCM. In view of the problems mentioned above in the development of TCM, Chairman Mao Zedong put forward three basic principles of health work in China: "Facing workers, peasants, and soldiers; giving priority to prevention, and integrating TCM and WM." These thoughts and measures promoted the development and progress of TCM and made important contributions to the vigorous development of TCM in China.

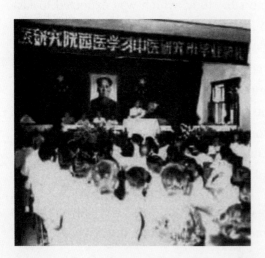

*In 1950, Chairman Mao Zedong wrote an inscription for the first National Health Work Conference, "Unite the medical and health staff from TCM and WM, old and new, form a solid united front, and strive for the great people's health work"*

*Graduation Ceremony of the First National Western Medicine Learning Traditional Chinese Medicine Class*

## II Using Scientific Methods to Study TCM—the Establishment of the Institute of Traditional Chinese Medicine

In 1950, at the first National Health Work Conference, the unity of Chinese and Western medicine was set as one of the essential policies of health work, which completely corrected the lingering thought of despising, discriminating against, and rejecting TCM. With the care and support of the Party and the government, TCM entered a brand-new stage of development. In June 1954, Chairman Mao Zedong instructed, "We need to immediately set up a TCM research institution, recruit brilliant TCM doctors to conduct research, send eminent WM doctors to study TCM, and participate in research work together." On October 26, 1954, the Party Group of the Culture and Education Committee of the State Council submitted to the Central Committee The Report on Improving the Work of Traditional Chinese Medicine. In the report, it was suggested "establish an Institute of Traditional Chinese Medicine" and its implementation was promptly approved by the Central Committee. From October 1954 to December 1955, after more than a year of intensive preparation, the Institute took over several units, such as the former Acupuncture and Moxibustion Experimental Institute of the Ministry of Health and basically completed the preparatory work for the construction of the Institute of Traditional Chinese Medicine.

On December 19, 1955, the Institute of Traditional Chinese Medicine of the Ministry of Health of the People's Republic of China's inaugural meeting was grandly held in the Beixian Pavilion of Guang'anmennei, Beijing. "Carry forward the medical heritage of the motherland and serve for the socialist construction", Premier Zhou Enlai personally wrote an inscription for the establishment of the Institute of Traditional Chinese Medicine. The Ministry of Health appointed Lu Zhijun as the first president of the Institute of Traditional Chinese Medicine, Zhu Lian and Tian Runzhi as vice presidents, Peng Zemin as honorary president, and Xiao Longyou as honorary vice president. On the same day, leaders such as Li Jishen, Xie Juezai, Xi Zhongxun, Xu Teli, and Zhang Jichun attended the meeting. About 400 people from relevant departments, such as the National Committee of the Chinese People's Political Consultative Conference, the United Front Work Department, the State Council, and the Ministry of Health, were invited to attend.

After the establishment of the Institute of Traditional Chinese Medicine, more than 30 famous TCM experts were selected from all over the country, and 8 institutes were established to carry out scientific research, clinical and educational work in internal medicine, surgery, gynecology and pediatrics, orthopedics, ophthalmology, acupuncture, and Chinese materia medica, which cultivated many senior talents for the development of TCM and promoted TCM to be an essential part of China's disease prevention and control forces. It ushered in a new era of scientific research on TCM.

The establishment of the Institute of Traditional Chinese Medicine marks the beginning of the scientific and organized study, collation, and improvement of the medical heritage of the motherland under the unified guidance of specialized institutions. After several generations of efforts, the Institute of Traditional Chinese Medicine was renamed China Academy of Chinese Medical Sciences (CACMS) in 2005 and developed into a state-level comprehensive TCM research institute integrating

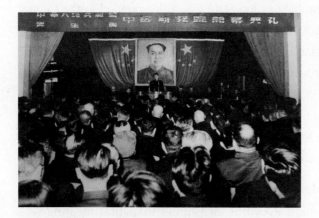

scientific research, medical treatment, education, and industry, leading the continuous development of TCM in China.

*The venue of the Inaugural Meeting of the Institute of Traditional Chinese Medicine, Ministry of Health of the People's Republic of China (1955)*

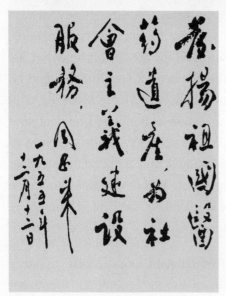

*In 1955, Premier Zhou Enlai wrote an inscription for the establishment of the Institute of Traditional Chinese Medicine*

## III TCM's Entry into the New Era of Independent Development—the Founding of the State Administration of Traditional Chinese Medicine

Before the birth of the State Administration of Traditional Chinese Medicine, there was no independent administrative organization of TCM in China, and the work of TCM was always managed by the Department of TCM of the Ministry of Health, which was always in a subordinate position in China's medical and health undertakings. In 1978, the work of Chinese materia medica was transferred from the health department to the State Administration of Medicine. Therefore, traditional Chinese medicine and Chinese materia medica were facing a state of "separation". Facing the severe problems in the management and development of TCM, the TCM community reacted strongly. In 1984, ten famous TCM experts, including He Ren, Zhang Canjia, and Li Jinyong, wrote to the State Council stating the severe institutional defects restricted the development of TCM, earnestly hoping to establish an independent TCM management system and the State Administration of Traditional Chinese Medicine. Hu Ximing, the former deputy minister of the Ministry of Health and the first director of the State Administration of Traditional Chinese Medicine, also pointed out that "if we want to carry forward TCM, we should implement independent management of TCM". The strong voices inside and outside the industry have aroused great attention from the CPC Central Committee.

The CPC Central Committee and the State Council discussed the issue of TCM 5 times. After in-depth investigation and research, on January 4, 1986, the 94th Executive Meeting of the State Council decided to establish the State Administration of Traditional Chinese Medicine. In this meeting, it was pointed out that "TCM should be placed in an important position. The integration of Chinese and Western medicine is correct, but TCM cannot be reformed with WM. WM should be developed, and so should TCM and TCM should not be regarded as a subordinate to WM". On July 20, 1986, the State Council officially issued the Notice on the Establishment of the State Administration of Traditional Chinese Medicine, which clearly stipulated that "the State Administration of Traditional Chinese Medicine is an institution directly under the State Council and is managed by the Ministry of Health. Its main task is to manage the cause of

TCM and the training of TCM talents, inherit and carry forward TCM, and serve for the construction of socialist health cause with Chinese characteristics and improvement of the health level of the Chinese people".

The establishment of the State Administration of Traditional Chinese Medicine shows that the Party and the government attach great importance to the development of TCM. Since then, TCM has entered a new period of independent development from its subordinate position in the past. The development policies and mechanisms of TCM have been continuously improved, the scientific research construction of TCM has been continuously strengthened, and the ability of TCM to prevent and treat diseases has been continuously improved. The cause of TCM has taken on a new stage of prosperity.

# IV World-Shaking TCM Battle against SARS

In the spring of 2003, a sudden SARS epidemic came quietly. It is the first severe infectious disease discovered by humans in the 21st century, which is menacing and unprepared. In mid-to-late February of 2003, the SARS epidemic was prevalent in some areas of Guangdong, spread in North China in early March, and continued to develop in mid-to-late April, posing a great threat to people's health and life safety.

Beijing was hit hard by SARS at that time. The epidemic was extremely severe, with 1,347 confirmed SARS cases, 1,358 suspected cases, and 66 deaths in Beijing, according to the statistics on April 29, 2003. At the same time, there was exciting news from Guangzhou. Under the guidance of the famous TCM expert Deng Tietao's theory of treating SARS, the First Affiliated Hospital of Guangzhou University of Chinese Medicine achieved a good record of zero death, sequelae, and nosocomial infection in patients treated; a total of 112 patients were treated in Guangdong Provincial Hospital of Chinese Medicine with a cure rate of more than 90%. The World Health Organization (WHO) visited the Guangdong Provincial Hospital of Chinese Medicine and spoke highly of the treatment of SARS with the integration of traditional Chinese and Western medicine on April 7. The SARS Leading Group of the Ministry of Health issued a notice on the Technical Scheme for the Prevention and Treatment of SARS with Traditional Chinese Medicine (Trial) on April 11, which clearly pointed out: "The practice of prevention and treatment of SARS in Guangdong Province shows that the method of combining traditional Chinese and Western medicine is better than that of Western medicine alone." On May 8, 2003, Ms Wu Yi, Vice Premier of the State Council and Minister of Health, held a symposium with well-known TCM experts in Beijing, emphasizing that TCM is an important force in fighting against SARS. The scientific value of TCM should be fully recognized, TCM resources should be actively utilized, the role of medical staff should be given full play, and the mission of prevention and treatment of SARS should be accomplished by integrating traditional Chinese and Western medicine. After this meeting, TCM officially entered the main battlefield of fighting against SARS in Beijing. Since May 11, Beijing has taken measures to ensure that all designated SARS hospitals have the participation of TCM. Most inpatients have been treated with integrated

Chinese and Western medicine, with noticeable effects. The epidemic in Beijing has been gradually brought under control. In early June, TCM experts were stationed at Xiaotangshan Hospital, further promoting the treatment program of integrated Chinese and Western medicine. On June 24, the WHO lifted its travel warning on Beijing and removed Beijing from the list of SARS epidemic areas with "recent local transmission", which marked a major victory in the prevention and treatment of SARS in China.

In October 2003, WHO and the National Administration of Traditional Chinese Medicine jointly held the International Symposium on Treating SARS with the Combination of Traditional Chinese Medicine and Western Medicine in Beijing. 17 international experts from WHO listened to the research report on the participation of TCM in the prevention and treatment of SARS. The experts at the meeting agreed that the combination of traditional Chinese and Western medicine in the treatment of SARS was safe and had potential benefits in many aspects, and spoke highly of the critical role of integrated Chinese and Western medicine in the treatment of SARS.

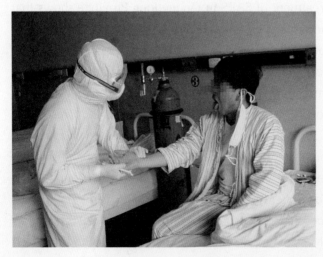

*TCM experts treating SARS*
*patients at Beijing Ditan Hospital*

## V The First Chinese Nobel Laureate in Physiology or Medicine—Tu Youyou

On October 5, 2015, the Nobel Prize in Physiology or Medicine winners was announced, and Chinese scientist Tu Youyou won the Nobel Prize for her outstanding contribution to the innovation of malaria therapy. This is the first time that a Chinese scientist has won the Nobel Prize for scientific research in China, and it is also the highest international award for medical achievements in China.

Tu Youyou was born in Ningbo, Zhejiang Province, in 1930. At 16, she was forced to terminate her studies for more than two years because of pulmonary tuberculosis. It was then that Tu Youyou, who was in high school, became interested in medicine. In 1951, she was admitted to the Pharmacy Department of Beijing Medical College (now Peking University Health Science Center). This "unpopular" major finally got her involved with TCM. After graduating from Beijing Medical College, Tu Youyou worked at the China Academy of Traditional Chinese Medicine (renamed China Academy of Chinese Medical Sciences in 2005). During her work, she attended the third training course on theories and practices of TCM, intended for professionals with a WM training background.

In the 1960s, chloroquine failed to fight against malaria, and human beings suffered from it. The China Academy of Traditional Chinese Medicine accepted the national malaria prevention and control project "523" anti-malaria research project in 1969. Facing this arduous task, Tu Youyou resolutely shouldered the heavy burden. Starting from the systematic collection of medical books, herbs and folk prescriptions of the past dynasties, she led the research group to compile *Collection of Single Prescription for Antimalarial Treatment* with 640 kinds of drugs and carried out experimental research on more than 200 kinds of Chinese medicines. After hundreds of experiments, she further digested the sentence "A handful of Qinghao immersed in 2 liters of water, wring out the juice and drink it all" in the *Handbook of Prescriptions for Emergency* when Qinghao was mentioned for alleviating the cold or heat malaria symptoms. The research group used modern medicine and methods to analyze, study, and constantly improve the extraction method. It was found that the neutral portion of the ether extract of *artemisia annua* could inhibit *malaria parasite* by up to 100%. After further isolation, in 1971, artemisinin, an antimalarial monomer effective in treating malaria was finally obtained. Since its introduction, it has saved millions of lives worldwide. On June 30, 2021, the WHO declared that China was certified as malaria-free, reducing the number of malaria infections in China from 30 million in the 1940s to zero. This is a remarkable achievement, and artemisinin has contributed significantly.

As Tu Youyou said, artemisinin is a gift from TCM to people worldwide. For decades, she and her team have never stopped exploring. She has built a bridge between TCM and modern medicine and also opened a door for all scientific researchers to go global.

# VI The Promulgation of China's First TCM Law

On December 25, 2016, the 25th session of the 12th National People's Congress (NPC) Standing Committee passed the *Law of the People's Republic of China on Traditional Chinese Medicine* (after this, referred to as the *TCM Law*), which marked the birth of China's first national law on the revitalization of TCM.

As early as 1983, Dong Jianhua, a deputy to the National People's Congress, put forward a motion to enact the law on TCM. Since then, at successive sessions of the National People's Congress and the National Committee of the Chinese People's Political Consultative Conference, there have been numerous motions and proposals on the legislation on TCM. In 1986, Li Peng, the then Premier of the State Council, ordered that a regulation on the revitalization of TCM should be developed first and that the legislation should be enacted when conditions were ripe. Subsequently, the State Council began drafting the *Regulations of the People's Republic of China on Traditional Chinese Medicine* (after this, referred to as the *Regulations*) and promulgated the *Regulations* in April 2003. With the continuous development of TCM in China, there are increasing strong voices inside and outside the industry expecting to formulate a TCM law based on the *Regulations*. According to the proposals of the Legislative Affairs Office of the State Council and the Ministry of Health on starting the drafting of TCM legislation, the National Administration of Traditional Chinese Medicine started drafting the TCM law in March 2005. After several drafts, the *Law of the People's Republic of China on Traditional Chinese Medicine* (draft) was formed in 2006. In October 2008, the *TCM Law* was included in the five-year legislative plan of the Standing Committee of the 11th National People's Congress. From 2008 to 2015, the National Administration of Traditional Chinese Medicine reorganized the drafting of the *TCM Law* and set up eight research groups across the country, divided into two large groups in the north and south. After several rounds of research and expert review, a new *TCM Law* (draft) was formulated, and submitted to the State Council by the Ministry of Health at the end of 2011. The Legislative Affairs Office of the State Council repeatedly solicited opinions from relevant departments of the central government, local governments, and some medical institutions, universities, as well as from experts, conducted nine field investigations in Beijing, Inner Mongolia, Guangdong, and Guizhou, solicited opinions from the public for many times, and constantly revised and improved the *TCM Law* (draft). Finally, it was deliberated by the Standing Committee of the National People's Congress in 2016 and officially promulgated by the presidential decree signed by President Xi.

As the first comprehensive law that comprehensively and systematically reflects the characteristics of TCM, the *TCM Law* codifies the Party's and state's guidelines and policies on the development of TCM in a legal form and embodies people's expectations and demands for TCM in a legal form, which shows that the Party and the state attach great importance to the cause of TCM and is of landmark significance for the development of the TCM industry.

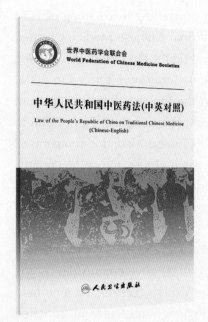

*Law of the People's Republic of China on Traditional Chinese Medicine (Chinese-English), published in 2017 by People's Medical Publishing House*

# VII Traditional Medicine's Official Enrollment into the International Classification of Diseases 11th Revision (ICD-11)

On May 25, 2019, the 72nd World Health Assembly reviewed and approved the International Classification of Diseases 11th Revision (ICD-11), which included a chapter on traditional medicine originating from TCM for the first time. This is a valuable achievement of the continuous efforts of the Chinese government and TCM experts over the past ten years.

The International Classification of Diseases (ICD) is an internationally unified classification standard of diseases formulated and promulgated by WHO. It is the normative standard for disease classification in the medical treatment, management, teaching, scientific research, and policy-making by governments of various countries, and it is also one of the authoritative foundations and universal standards in the field of global health. After WHO started the 11th revision of the ICD in 2007, the National Administration of Traditional Chinese Medicine organized the national TCM experts for discussion and demonstration. In 2009, entrusted by the National Administration of Traditional Chinese Medicine, the Shanghai Traditional Chinese Medicine Development Office (now Shanghai Municipal Administrator of Traditional Chinese Medicine) assumed the project management responsibility. Academician Zhang Boli and Professor Yan Shiyun of Shanghai University of Traditional Chinese Medicine led a team of 36 project review experts. Nearly 100 experts from all over the country formed various technical groups on terminology, information, standards, and classification. Under the leading organization and technical guidance of WHO, through long-term efforts, and finally through the cooperation of China and relevant countries to seek common ground while reserving differences, the supplementary chapter on traditional medicine was included in Chapter 26 of ICD-11. The traditional medicine diseases and syndromes that originated in ancient China and are currently widely used in China, Japan, Korea, and other countries have been classified and named as "Supplementary Chapter Traditional Medicine Conditions-Module I", including 150 traditional medicine diseases and 196 syndromes (excluding specific and non-specific diseases and syndromes). In this chapter, TCM diagnosis is coded according to disease name (disorders) and patterns, such as jaundice, and its code is SA01, and qi deficiency pattern and its code are SE90. Each disease can be defined by its symptoms, etiology, course, and outcome or treatment response.

After traditional medicine originating from TCM was covered in ICD-11, it can be popularized and disseminated simultaneously with the ICD system to form an international standardized language of TCM disease and syndrome classification system, promote the formation of international consensus of TCM in clinical, scientific research, education, management, insurance, and other fields, enhance the integrity, scientificity, and universality of statistical information of TCM services, and help promote the development of TCM international medical services.

## VIII Inherit the Essence, Maintain Integrity and Innovate— Comprehensively Promote the Revitalization and Development of TCM

Since the 18th CPC National Congress in 2012, China regards the inheritance, innovation, and development of TCM as a major event for the great rejuvenation of the Chinese nation. In 2016, the Outline of the Strategic Plan on the Development of Traditional Chinese Medicine (2016–2030) was released, and the development of TCM was elevated to a national strategy. In 2017, the promulgation of The law of the People's Republic of China on Traditional Chinese Medicine provided legal protection for the development of TCM. In October 2019, the Opinions of the Central Committee of the Communist Party of China and the State Council on Promoting the Inheritance, Innovation and Development of Traditional Chinese Medicine was issued, and the State Council held the National Conference on Traditional Chinese Medicine, which raised the whole society's understanding of TCM to an unprecedented level. In 2022, the 14th Five-Year Plan for the Development of Traditional Chinese Medicine was issued, which made a comprehensive, strategic, and supportive plan for the development of TCM. The report of the 20th CPC National Congress proposed to promote the inheritance, innovation, and development of TCM, which further pointed out the direction for the high-quality development of TCM in the new era.

With the guidance of national strategy, TCM is fully integrated into the Healthy China Action. The service capacity of TCM has been further improved, the construction of talent team has been further strengthened, the inheritance work has been continuously promoted, and new breakthroughs have been made in scientific and technological innovation. The development of TCM has yielded fruitful results, and has written one brilliant chapter after another in practice. In 2019, the first batch of national clinical medical research centers in the field of TCM were approved; in the same year, the world's first evidence-based medicine center in the field of TCM was established at the China Academy of Chinese Medical Sciences (CACMS). In 2020, the Fourth National Survey of Traditional Chinese Medicine Resources was completed, which obtained over 2 million survey records and summarized information on the types and distribution of over 13,000 types of traditional Chinese medicine resources. In 2021, A neuroanatomical basis for electroacupuncture to drive the vagal—adrenal axis, completed by Professor Ma Qiufu of Harvard Medical School, Professor Wang Yanqing of Fudan University, and Professor Jing Xianghong of the Acupuncture and Moxibustion Research Institute of CACMS, was published in *Nature*, a top international journal. In 2022, the China Administration of Traditional Chinese Medicine took the lead in formulating the policy document Opinions on Strengthening the Work of Traditional Chinese Medicine Talents in the New Era for the first time. In 2023, after 11 years, the first batch of books of *The Chinese Medical Collection* compiled by nearly a thousand people from 28 institutions and 34 research groups across the country were released in The National Library of China.

TCM embodies the health and wellness concepts and practical experience of the Chinese nation for thousands of years, and embodies the vast wisdom of the Chinese people and the Chinese nation. Only by inheriting the essence can TCM achieve sustainable development; only by adhering to integrity and innovation can we inject a continuous stream of vitality into the development of TCM. At a new historical starting point, inheriting the essence, upholding integrity and innovation will surely make TCM obtain infinite vitality, contribute to the construction of a healthy China, and play a greater role in building a community with a shared future for mankind.